Head and Neck Oncology

Head and Neck Oncology

A Concise Guide

Edited by

Dr. Akheel Mohammad
MDS, MFDS RCPS (Glasg), FDS RCS (Lon), FHNCS, FIFHNOS (US), (PhD)
Consultant Head & Neck Oncosurgeon/Reconstruction Surgeon
Indore, India

Dr. Ashmi Wadhwania
MDS, PGDEMS
Consultant Oral & Maxillofacial Surgeon
Indore, India

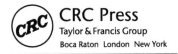

CRC Press
Taylor & Francis Group
Boca Raton London New York

CRC Press is an imprint of the
Taylor & Francis Group, an **informa** business

First edition published 2022
by CRC Press
6000 Broken Sound Parkway NW, Suite 300, Boca Raton, FL 33487-2742
and by CRC Press
2 Park Square, Milton Park, Abingdon, Oxon, OX14 4RN

© 2022 Taylor & Francis Group, LLC
CRC Press is an imprint of Taylor & Francis Group, LLC

ISBN: 9780367640972 (hbk)
ISBN: 9780367421311 (pbk)
ISBN: 9780367822019 (ebk)

DOI: 10.1201/9780367822019

Typeset in Times LT Std
by KnowledgeWorks Global Ltd.

DEDICATED

TO

ALMIGHTY ALLAH

MY PARENTS,

MY LIFE PARTNER

MY TEACHERS

&

MY BELOVED FRIENDS

I dedicate this book to all my head/neck cancer patients and cancer survivors who have fought continuously and won the battle against this deadly disease with their extraordinary willpower, strength and patience.

I also dedicate this book to all those family members of these patients who have provided their constant support and complete cooperation with us for completion of the treatment.

We all must salute these patients for placing their trust in us and for bearing all the psychological and physical pain they have suffered during their treatment.

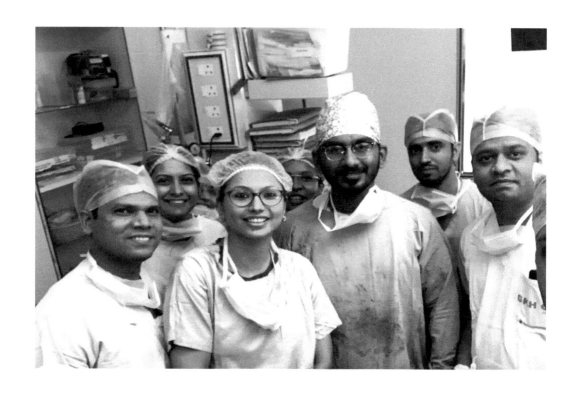

This book was written and structured to its form during the pandemic

COVID-19 that hit almost 200 countries across the globe. We pray

to ALMIGHTY GOD to shower blessings on us.

Contents

Foreword

By Dr. Jatin P. Shah

The specialty of head and neck surgery was developed simply as a subspecialty of "Cancer Surgery" in the post-war era of the 20th century. Radical operations became a hallmark for surgical treatment of neoplasms in the head and neck. The success of these surgical procedures was fueled by the availability of safe anesthesia, blood transfusions and antibiotics. This enthusiasm in radical surgery was introduced largely due to failure of radiotherapy alone in the treatment of head and neck tumors. However, despite the seeming success of radical surgery, local/regional failures were observed in a significant number of patients. Combining surgery with radiotherapy improved locoregional control and ushered in the concept of multimodal treatments. Introduction of cytotoxic chemotherapy for solid tumors in the second half of the 20th century added further armamentarium in the treatment of head and neck cancer, and the concept of organ preservation took center stage. By now, the specialty had evolved into "Head and Neck Surgery and Oncology", a truly multidisciplinary specialty. Advances in technology, molecular biology, genomics, pharmacology and identification of targets at the cellular level gave a further boost to therapeutics, with increasing emphasis on function, esthetics and quality of life.

Dr. Akheel Mohammad and Dr. Ashmi Wadhwania have crystalized a whole plethora of literature in the specialty and put together a very concise and user-friendly "Handbook" aimed at young trainees and even practitioners involved in the care of patients with head and neck cancer. According to the authors, the book is written along the guidelines of National Comprehensive Cancer Network (NCCN). These are merged with the experience of the authors in the workup and therapeutic strategies recommended for various tumors. Presentation of details in a "bullet list" fashion is visually appealing and makes it an easy read. This handbook is an excellent "introduction" to the specialty of head and neck surgery and oncology and readily meets the needs of a beginner in the field. Clearly, the authors have succeeded in their goal to offer a "Concise Guide in Head and Neck Oncology".

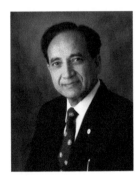

Dr. Jatin P. Shah, MD, PhD (Hon), DSc (Hon), FACS, FRCS (Hon),
FDSRCS (Hon), FRCSDS (Hon), FRCSI (Hon), FRACS (Hon)
Professor of Surgery
E W Strong Chair in Head and Neck Oncology
Memorial Sloan Kettering Cancer Center
New York, NY

Foreword

By Ashok R. Shaha

It is indeed a great honor and special pleasure for me to write this Foreword for *Head and Neck Oncology: A Concise Guide*, the book authored by Dr. Mohammad Akheel and Dr. Ashmi Wadhwania. Head and neck cancer continue to be a major problem around the world and especially in India. The goals of the treatment should be best cancer control, appropriate functional rehabilitation and cosmetic concerns. The management of head and neck cancer is a complex issue best planned by the head and neck multidisciplinary team. Even though there are several books published on this subject, Dr. Akheel's book is quite different as a concise guide to the management of head and neck cancer. It is amazing to see a two-authored book while the majority of the books today are authored by several physicians and compiled together by an editor. Dr. Akheel and Dr. Wadhwania have done a remarkable job in preparing this book with 26 chapters on various aspects of head and neck tumors. They have included subjects like carcinogenesis, molecular biology, staging and tumors of the specific organ sites. They have also included chapters on pain management and perioperative care. This is a remarkable undertaking, and I would like to congratulate both the authors for this handy book for trainees and a source of information for practicing head and neck oncologists. The book is easy to read and provides the appropriate direction to the understanding of this complex subject. I am sure this will be a ready reference for everyone involved in head and neck oncology. I wish the very best. Stay safe and God bless.

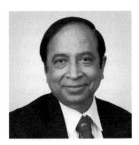

Ashok R. Shaha, MD
Professor of Surgery
Head and Neck Service
Memorial Sloan Kettering Cancer Center
New York, NY

A Note from the Editor

"OPERATING ROOM AND PATHOLOGICAL LABORATORY MUST BE A BRIDGE BUT NOT A GULF"

"FRIENDSHIP OF AN ONCOSURGEON WITH AN ONCOPATHOLOGIST IS MANDATORY"

The friendship between an oncosurgeon and an oncopathologist is something that is important if the primary objective of the surgery is to be addressed. Performing a biopsy from a suitable area and maximum clinical activity for diagnosis are important to solve the purpose of the procedure. Usually, these procedures are performed by an assistant; the oncosurgeon must personally perform this procedure due to its utmost importance to communicate with the oncopathologist regarding the facts and history of the patient. This sample must be properly oriented and a complete history must be documented in order for the pathologist understand the provisional clinical diagnosis. An inconclusive report from a pathologist can change the whole scenario and land the surgeon and pathologist in trouble, thereby having to repeat the biopsy.

It is an era of frozen section, which is most commonly used in developed countries for some inaccessible anatomical areas rather than conventional biopsy techniques. Urgency of the situation must also be taken in consideration. The paraffin sections take a minimum of 48 hours and can depend upon the number of reports to be addressed in contrast to the frozen section that can be done intraoperatively within 30 minutes with more precision and gives a realistic assessment in planning of the surgeon at the same time. Frozen sections can also be used during the surgery where the margins are still in doubt, but the extent to which it is used to establish the margin of clearance varies from surgeon to surgeon.

Systematic orientation of the specimen (anterior margin, posterior margin, superior margin, inferior margins and base, all lymph node levels) after the surgery with documentation is required and mandatory for proper understanding of the oncopathologist. This specimen must be placed in a proper fixation liquid like normal saline or formalin, 10 times more than that of the specimen to the pathologist to prevent distortion. Shrinkage of margins is 40–50%, which must be taken in to consideration by a surgeon. The final histopathology report is the key to deciding the patient or the surgeon's fate and role of adjuvant of therapies.

Adequacy and clearance are the two important points to deciding the prognosis of the patient based on the report. If the surgeon is not happy with the pathologist's competence, it is his choice to approach the other well-experienced pathologist, but at the same time, the surgeon must provide all the data and clear the doubts of the pathologist when required. There tends to be a gulf between the operating room and pathological laboratory, which is more than merely geographical. This gulf can be bridged properly when a surgeon and a pathologist, by performing their duties properly and sincerely, spend some time on every case, and it's an obvious fact that this relationship is built on a foundation of mutual respect and fostered by constant communication to improve the prognosis and overall survival of a patient.

Dr. Akheel Mohammad

Preface

The current population of India is 1.3 billion and still counting. Head and neck cancers account for one-third of all the cancer cases in India. According to the Indian Council of Medical Research (ICMR), 0.2–0.3 million new head and neck cancer patients are diagnosed every year in India. There are around 27 regional cancer centers in India with no centralized system to deal with head and neck cancer patients. Every center has its own institutional protocol different from the others to treat the same-stage patients. This concise handbook is a guide that is unique in its own kind, covering all important aspects of head and neck cancer. We have tried to cover all information required from basic topics like carcinogenesis to advanced treatment options like immunotherapy, electrochemotherapy and robotic surgery for head and neck cancers.

The management of cancers of all anatomic areas is written according to National Comprehensive Cancer Network (NCCN) guidelines V.2.2019, which is the workhorse in protocol for management of cancers, and every head and neck oncosurgeon must be aware of these guidelines. This book will serve as a valuable guide to postgraduate residents of maxillofacial surgery, ENT and otolaryngology, general surgery, plastic surgery and also junior specialists who are working in the field of head and neck oncology for diagnosis and systematically planning the treatment of the patient. We hope our readers will feel the inspired raptures after reading this book.

Dr. Akheel Mohammad

Acknowledgments

I am very thankful to Almighty GOD for instilling the idea of writing of this book and helping me in all my endeavors.

I am very thankful and obliged to my father, Mohammad Hameed, my mother, Tahera Sultana, and my brother, Mohammad Afroz, who were always there as my support, and whatever I am now is because of their prayers, love and affection.

I am very thankful to my coauthor, my inspiration and my beloved life partner Dr. Ashmi Wadhwania, a gorgeous maxillofacial surgeon and my head and neck team member, without whose help and contribution, this book might have not been possible.

I sincerely thank my fellowship guides Dr. Raj Nagarkar (Chairman and Surgical Oncologist) and Dr. Sirshendu Roy (Surgical Oncologist) of the HCG Curie Manavata Cancer Centre, Nasik, India, for giving me the opportunity to learn and pursue oncology as my career and thereby making my dream come true.

I sincerely thank my postgraduate and undergraduate teachers who have taught me; academics and discipline are two important things in life which make a man successful in his career.

I am thankful to all my friends and well-wishers who are always there motivating me during my bad times.

1

Carcinogenesis

Carcinogenesis is the process of induction of tumor and the agents that induce these tumors are called carcinogens. Carcinogens are broadly classified into

1. Chemical carcinogens
2. Physical carcinogens
3. Hormonal carcinogens
4. Biological carcinogens

Chemical Carcinogens

The first report of any chemical-causing neoplasia came from the observation in 1775 that there was a higher incidence of scrotum cancer in chimney sweepers in London than in the general population (Flowcharts 1.1 and 1.2).

Induction of cancer by chemical carcinogens can occur after delay of weeks to months or even years after exposure

↓

Induction depends on dose and mode of administration of carcinogenic chemical, individual susceptibility and other factors.

↓

Initiation

FLOWCHART 1.1   Initiation of carcinogenesis.

A single dose of an initiating agent for a large duration is more effective than a short dose with frequent exposure:

- *Direct-acting carcinogens*: Alkylating agents/acylating agents
- *Indirect-acting carcinogens*: Polycyclic aromatic hydrocarbons (tobacco)/azodyes

DOI: 10.1201/9780367822019-1

Mechanism:

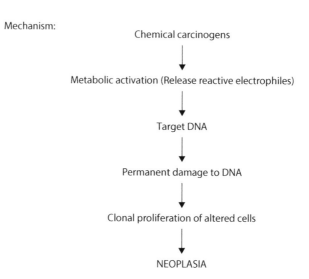

Chemical carcinogens

↓

Metabolic activation (Release reactive electrophiles)

↓

Target DNA

↓

Permanent damage to DNA

↓

Clonal proliferation of altered cells

↓

NEOPLASIA

FLOWCHART 1.2   Mechanism of carcinogenesis.

Physical Carcinogenesis

Physical causes are divided into

1. *Radiation agents*: UV light, ionizing radiation
2. *Non-radiation agents*

UV light: The main source of UV radiation is sunlight. It usually penetrates the skin for a few millimeters so that its effect is limited to epidermis. Excessive exposure can cause various forms of skin cancers, such as basal cell carcinoma, keratoacanthoma, and malignant melanoma.

Ionizing radiation: This includes all kinds such as X-rays, radioactive isotopes, protons, and neutrons. The most frequent radiation-induced cancers are leukemia, thyroid cancers, skin cancers, and salivary gland tumors.

Hormonal Carcinogenesis

Cancer is more often seen to develop in organs that undergo proliferation under the influence of excessive stimulation of hormones. Hormone-sensitive tissues that develop tumors are the breast, endometrium, vagina, prostate, and testis.

Biological Carcinogenesis

Biological carcinogenesis has been studied that about 20% of all cancers worldwide are viral-associated cancers. Sanarelli, an Italian physician, in 1889 was the first person who observed the association of oncogenic viruses with the neoplasia.

Examples include DNA oncovirus: Human papillomavirus/Epstein-Barr virus/cytomegalovirus/herpes simplex virus. RNA oncovirus: Human T-cell lymphotropic virus (HTLV).

Theories of Carcinogenesis

Important information:

1. *Proto-oncogenes:* These are normal genes that bring about cellular differentiation and growth. They can be converted into oncogenes.
2. *Oncogenes:* These are genes associated with neoplastic transformation.
3. *Anti-oncogenes:* These are cells that normally suppress cell proliferation. They are also called tumor suppressor genes.

Cancer may arise not only by activation of proto-oncogenes into oncogenes but also by suppressor of anti-oncogenes.

The following sections discuss the theories of carcinogenesis.

Genetic Theory

Genetic theory is the most popular and accepted theory. This theory suggests that the cells become neoplastic due to alterations in the DNA. The mutated cell transmits its character to the next progeny.

Epigenetic Theory

According to epigenetic theory, carcinogenic agents act on the activators or suppressors of genes and not on the gene themselves, which results in the abnormal expression of genes.

Multistep Theory

Carcinogenesis is a multistep process. This is substantiated by in vitro changes in the experimental animals as well as in vivo changes in human cancers.

For example, in chemical carcinogenesis, two essential features occur in proper sequence—initiation and promotion.

Most cancers arise after several mutations, which have been acquired in proper sequential manner.

Immune Surveillance Theory

An immune-competent host often mounts an attack on developing tumor cells to destroy them, while an immune incompetent host fails to destroy them. Some evidence in support of this theory is the fact that there is a high incidence of cancer in AIDS patients and most cancers occur in old people, where the host immune response is weak.

Monoclonal Theory

This theory suggests that cancers arise from a single clone of transformed cells.

Tumor Heterogeneity

This theory by Fidler and Ellis[1] states that a tumor is composed of subpopulations heterogeneous of cells. They will differ with respect to their immunogenicity, invasiveness, and sensitivity to cytotoxic drugs. But the environment of local tumor cells may favor the expansion of more aggressive clone information of metastasis (Flowcharts 1.3 and 1.4).

MYERS MODEL:

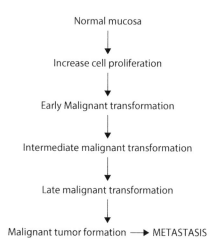

Normal mucosa

↓

Increase cell proliferation

↓

Early Malignant transformation

↓

Intermediate malignant transformation

↓

Late malignant transformation

↓

Malignant tumor formation ⟶ METASTASIS

FLOWCHART 1.3   Myers model.

STEPS IN CARCINOGENESIS:

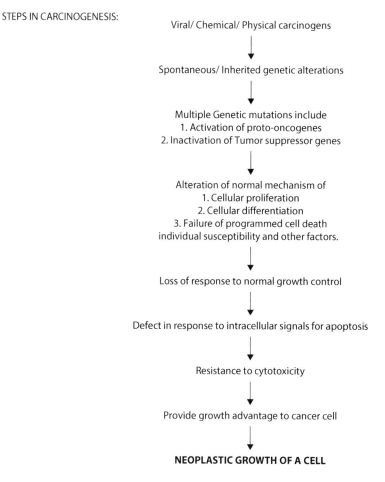

Viral/ Chemical/ Physical carcinogens

↓

Spontaneous/ Inherited genetic alterations

↓

Multiple Genetic mutations include
1. Activation of proto-oncogenes
2. Inactivation of Tumor suppressor genes

↓

Alteration of normal mechanism of
1. Cellular proliferation
2. Cellular differentiation
3. Failure of programmed cell death
individual susceptibility and other factors.

↓

Loss of response to normal growth control

↓

Defect in response to intracellular signals for apoptosis

↓

Resistance to cytotoxicity

↓

Provide growth advantage to cancer cell

↓

NEOPLASTIC GROWTH OF A CELL

FLOWCHART 1.4   Steps in carcinogenesis.

Field Cancerization

Secondary tumors of the oral cavity have a sobering effect on the prognosis for head and neck cancer (HNC) patients. These tumors are most often seen to develop in the oral cavity but can also be seen in lungs or esophagus from which 10–40% of patients with HNC are often fatal. One of the reasons for this multifocal tumor origin was proposed around 40 years ago by Slaughter et al. In accordance with his concept of field cancerization, there are multiple cell groups that independently undergo neoplastic transformation due to stress of regional carcinogenic activity. There are certain molecular genetic approaches that have been recently challenged with the fact that independent transforming events are more common in the epithelial mucosa of HNC patients. Often, when a primary cancer is compared with a secondary tumor somewhere in oral cavity/upper aerodigestive tract, these paired tumors often harbor cells that have identical patterns of genetic alterations or mutations. It is assumed that single cell regimens a critical genetic for advantage of growth over its neighboring cells. At some point of time after the transformation, cells which harbor these early genetic alterations then migrate to nearby adjacent areas to populate contiguous tracts of mucosa further accumulating other alterations that later acquire additional growth advantages from the surrounding environment, and ultimately transform into aggressive subclones that may be separated by space and time.

Secondly, collective observations have supported the view that the epithelial mucosa of the upper aerodigestive tract may become populated by these genetically damaged clones of cells, which may lack any histopathological evidence of dysplastic features. The presence of these genetically damaged but morphologically intact cells not only explains the phenomenon of field cancerization but also accounts for certain altered/distressing behavioral patterns of tumors, such as recurrence of tumor locally following macroscopically complete surgical resection. A lack of confidence growing among the pathologist's ability to recognize the extent and presence of the neoplastic process in patients who are at risk for cancer has accelerated a search of a novel biomarkers in the recognition and management of HNC.

Review of Literature

Hashibe et al. have extensively performed a study on the carcinogenesis in the area of the head and neck (H&N) use of tobacco and alcohol in humans. In this study, at least 75% of HNCs in Europe, the United States, and a few other industrialized and developed nations are exposed to the combinations of tobacco and alcohol use[2].

Wyss et al. studied risk of oral cancer associated with tobacco-related products and their variants. For combustible products, the study revealed increased risks of oral and oropharyngeal cancers for cigars (OR = 2.54, CI = 1.93–3.34), cigarettes (OR = 3.46, 95% CI = 3.24–3.70), cigars (OR = 2.54, CI = 1.93–3.34), and pipes (OR = 2.08, CI = 1.55–2.81)[2]. With respect to smokeless tobacco, the use of snuff has been associated with HNCs (OR = 1.71, CI = 1.08–2.70), particularly for oral cavity cancers (OR = 3.01, CI = 1.63–5.55), when confined to cancers of oral cavity, tobacco chewing had a very strong association (OR = 1.81, CI = 1.04–3.17)[3]. Moreover, while human papillomavirus (HPV)-induced oral and oropharyngeal cancer is increasing in incidence. A study of around 100,000 patients in 2013 showed that 66% of diagnosed HN squamous cell carcinoma (HNSCC) were alcohol and tobacco related[3]. Thus, tobacco remains a major reason of HNSCC.

Another study about the synergistic effect of alcohol and tobacco is supported by pooled data analysis from 17 American and European studies[4]. The population attributable risk for HNCs was 72%, which included 35% attributable to both alcohol and tobacco, 4% for alcohol alone, 33% for tobacco alone. The odds ratios for developing HNSCC are 2.37 (1.66–3.39) for people who use tobacco but do not use alcohol, 1.06 (0.88–1.28) for alcohol users who never use tobacco, and 5.73 (3.62–9.06) for people who use both alcohol and tobacco[5]. This synergistic effect was more than multiplicative. Dal Maso et al. demonstrated similar steep increases in the risk of HNSCC among tobacco and alcohol users, especially those users using high amounts of each product[6].

Koyanagi et al. identified 12 case control studies and 5 cohort studies. Of these 5 cohort studies, 4 cohort studies and 11 of 12 case control studies showed a strong positive association among HNC and smoking of cigarettes. Nine of the 12 studies indicated a dose–response relationship between cigarette smoking and the risk of HNCs. Meta-analysis of 12 studies summarized that the relative risk for people who had ever smoked compared to those who has never smoked was 2.43 (95% CI = 2.09–2.83). The relative risks for current and former smokers compared to never smokers were 2.68 (2.08–3.44) and 1.49 (1.05–2.11), respectively[7].

REFERENCES

1. Fidler IJ, Ellis LM. The implications of angiogenesis for the biology and therapy of cancer metastasis. *Cell.* 1994 Oct 21;79(2):185–8.
2. Hashibe M, Brennan P, Benhamou S, Castellsague X, Chen C, Curado MP, Maso LD, Daudt AW, Fabianova E, Wünsch-Filho V, Franceschi S. Alcohol drinking in never users of tobacco, cigarette smoking in never drinkers, and the risk of head and neck cancer: pooled analysis in the International Head and Neck Cancer Epidemiology Consortium. *Journal of the National Cancer Institute.* 2007 May 16;99(10):777–89.
3. Wyss A, Hashibe M, Chuang SC, Lee YC, Zhang ZF, Yu GP, Winn DM, Wei Q, Talamini R, Szeszenia-Dabrowska N, Sturgis EM. Cigarette, cigar, and pipe smoking and the risk of head and neck cancers: pooled analysis in the International Head and Neck Cancer Epidemiology Consortium. *American Journal of Epidemiology.* 2013 Sep 1;178(5):679–90.
4. Hashibe M, Hunt J, Wei M, Buys S, Gren L, Lee YC. Tobacco, alcohol, body mass index, physical activity, and the risk of head and neck cancer in the prostate, lung, colorectal, and ovarian (PLCO) cohort. *Head & Neck.* 2013 Jul;35(7):914–22.
5. Hashibe M, Brennan P, Chuang SC, Boccia S, Castellsague X, Chen C, Curado MP, Dal Maso L, Daudt AW, Fabianova E, Fernandez L. Interaction between tobacco and alcohol use and the risk of head and neck cancer: pooled analysis in the International Head and Neck Cancer Epidemiology Consortium. *Cancer Epidemiology, Biomarkers & Prevention.* 2009 Feb 1;18(2):541–50.
6. Dal Maso L, Torelli N, Biancotto E, Di Maso M, Gini A, Franchin G, Levi F, La Vecchia C, Serraino D, Polesel J. Combined effect of tobacco smoking and alcohol drinking in the risk of head and neck cancers: a re-analysis of case–control studies using bi-dimensional spline models. *European Journal of Epidemiology.* 2016 Apr 1;31(4):385–93.
7. Koyanagi YN, Matsuo K, Ito H, Wakai K, Nagata C, Nakayama T, Sadakane A, Tanaka K, Tamakoshi A, Sugawara Y, Mizoue T. Cigarette smoking and the risk of head and neck cancer in the Japanese population: a systematic review and meta-analysis. *Japanese Journal of Clinical Oncology.* 2016 Jun 1;46(6):580–95.

2

Molecular Biology of Cancer and Biomarkers

Cancer is a multifactorial disease with etiological agents being chemical, physical and biologic carcinogens. These lead to cancer as a result of alterations in cellular growth control process together with changes in the interaction between cells and their surroundings which gives rise to invasion and metastasis (Flowchart 2.1).

Recent evidence suggests 6–10 genetic events are required for development of oral cancer. At least four groups of genes are involved in this process, which include

1. Proto-oncogenes
2. Tumor suppressor genes
3. DNA repair genes
4. Sequences that control apoptosis

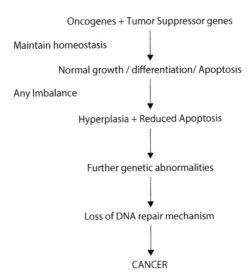

FLOWCHART 2.1 Activation of oncogenes and tumor suppressor genes that cause cancer.

Oncogenes and tumor suppressor genes together maintain homeostasis in the cell. They control activities like normal cellular growth, cellular differentiation and apoptosis. Any imbalance in these cells will lead to hyperplasia and reduced apoptosis. Further genetic abnormalities will lead to loss of DNA repair mechanism which causes uncontrolled proliferation of mutated cell leading to cancer.

Normal Cell Cycle

To understand the biology of cancer at a cellular level, understanding of the normal cell cycle is mandatory.

DOI: 10.1201/9780367822019-2

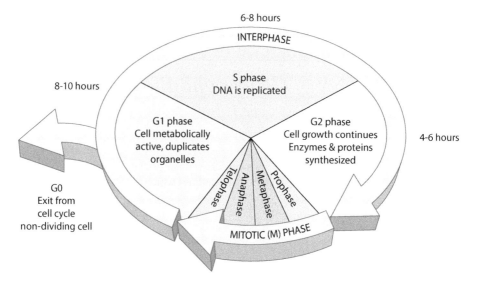

FIGURE 2.1   Cell cycle.

The **cell cycle** is nothing but the life cycle of a cell. In different words, it is a sequence of events of growth and development a single cell which undergoes between its "birth"—formation from the division of a mother cell until the reproduction—division of this cell to make two new daughter cells (Figure 2.1).

Stages of the Cell Cycle

For division, there are several important tasks to be completed by a cell: it must grow, duplicate its own genetic material called deoxyribonucleic acid, and eventually must split into two new daughter cells. Cells perform all these tasks in an organized and predictable fashion of steps that can collectively make up the cycle of cell. The cell cycle is an organized cycle, rather than a linear pathway, because each process produces two new cells that can repeat the process.

Eukaryotic cells have a nucleus and the stages of cell cycle are divided into two major phases, **interphase** and the **mitotic (M) phase**.

- During *interphase*, the cell grows and duplicates its DNA.
- During *mitotic (M) phase*, the cell separates its single DNA into two sets and then divides its cytoplasm and forms two new daughter cells.

Interphase

Let's study the cell cycle: How a cell forms, from the division of its mother cell. What is the mode of action of this new cell which is born and divides itself into two?

- *G1 phase*: This is also known as the first gap phase, during this phase the cell grows larger and makes more of its contents like organelles, ribosomes, and proteins. This phase confirms that division will produce functional daughter cells, which have the right size and have all the organelles they need. If cells don't grow well before they divide, they would get smaller and eventually become too small to function properly. G1 phase begins when a cell is "born" that is by division of its mother cell and ends with the onset of the next phase called S phase. G1 is the longest phase of the cell cycle in many cells.

- *S phase*: In order to divide, a cell also needs to duplicate its genetic material, allowing it to give one complete set of material to each of its own two daughter cells. For completion of this, the cell moves from G1 into a phase called S phase which synthesizes a complete copy of the DNA in its nucleus. During this phase, the cell also duplicates in a microtubule organizing structure called the centrosome. The two centrosomes play a key role in separating the DNA during M phase.
- *G2 phase*: Once synthesis of the DNA is complete, the cell then enters a second gap, which is called the G2 phase. During this phase, the cell further grows more and makes some additional organelles and proteins, and then begins to reorganize its contents for the preparation of mitosis, the separation of their copied DNA into two new equal sets. When mitosis begins, the G2 phase ends.

The G1, S, and G2 phases together are called the **interphase**. The prefix *inter* means between, reflecting that the interphase takes place between the two mitotic (M) phases.

M Phase

The interphase alternates with the mitotic (M) phase. During this M phase, the cell further divides its copied nuclear DNA and cytoplasm to form two new daughter cells. The M phase is divided further into two more phases: **mitosis** and **cytokinesis**.

In the mitotic phase, the nuclear DNA of the cell condenses into visible chromosomes and is pulled apart by the mitotic spindle, a specialized structure made out of microtubules. Mitosis takes place in four stages: the prophase (often divided into early prophase and prometaphase), metaphase, anaphase, and telophase.

G0 Phase

In the G0 phase, a cell does not actively divide, it just carries out its job. For instance, it might conduct signals as a neuron or store carbohydrates as a liver cell. Some cells, like neurons, permanently exit the cell cycle and remain in the G0 phase until they die.

Cell Cycle Checkpoints

Each checkpoint in a cell cycle serves as a potential point, during which the cell conditions are evaluated. When favorable conditions are met, transmission occurs through all the phases of the cell cycle. Presently, there are three known checkpoints: the G1 checkpoint that is also called the start checkpoint or restriction or major checkpoint, the G2/M checkpoint, and the metaphase checkpoint, also known as the spindle checkpoint (Figure 2.2).

G1 Checkpoint

The G1 checkpoint is also called the restriction of point in mammalian cells and the start point in yeast. It is defined as the point at which the cell gets committed to enter the cycle. As the cell continues to progress through G1 phase, depending on conditions externally and internally, it can either delay G1 checkpoint or enter a silent state known as G0 *phase* or it may proceed past the point of restriction. The decision to enter a new round of division of cell normally occurs when the cell activates cyclin-CDK-dependent transcription that promotes the entry of a cell into S phase.

G2 Checkpoint

After the division of cell, each cell enters the cycle and multiplies, and then goes through S phase, where it replicates its own DNA, G2 phase, and it then undergoes rapid synthesis and growth of protein in preparation for mitotic cell division. The G2/M checkpoint, also called the DNA damage checkpoint, confirms that the cell has undergone all of the changes necessary during the S and G2 phases and which are ready for division. Cyclin B-cdc2 complex is the primary complex responsible for the transition.

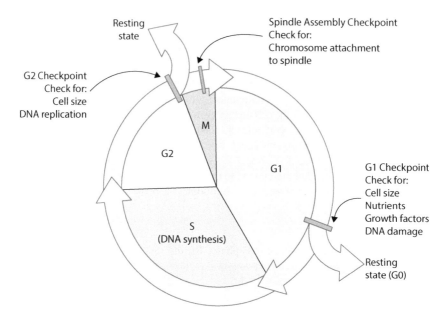

FIGURE 2.2   Cell cycle checkpoints.

Metaphase Checkpoint

The mitotic spindle checkpoint often occurs in the metaphase where the mitotic plate ensures that all the chromosomes are aligned under bipolar tension. This tension is created by this bipolar attachment which initiates the entry in to the anaphase. For this to happen, the sensing mechanism ensures that the promoting complex of *anaphase* is no longer inhibited, which is now free to degrade cyclin B, which now harbors a destruction box called D-box and breaks these securins. Securin is a protein, the function of which is to inhibit separase, which later cuts the cohesins. *Cohesin* is a protein composite which is responsible for sister chromatids cohesion. Once the degradation of inhibitory protein is done via ubiquitination process and subsequent proteolysis, separase then causes separation of sister chromatids. After the cell has split into its two daughter cells, the cell then enters the G1 phase.

Oncogenes

Oncogenes better termed as proto-oncogenes are derived from genetic material in each normal cell and play a pivotal role in growth and maturation of cells.

> *Carcinogen exposure causes consequent mutations which activates proto-oncogenes into oncogenes leading to formation of a tumor.*

There are four types of oncogenes: (1) growth factors like PDGF, (2) secondary messengers like H-ras, N-ras, etc., (3) gene transcriptions like "fas" and "jun" oncogenes, and (4) apoptosis regulators like Bcl-1, Bcl-2.

1. *Growth factors*: Some oncogenes encode growth factors, the molecules that initiate the signals for cell division. Growth factors like platelet-derived growth factors (PDGFs) are produced.
2. *Secondary messengers*: A group of oncogenes act to couple extracellular signals to cytoplasmic signaling mechanisms and are termed second messengers.
   - The "ras" gene is a member of this group. Examples include K-ras, H-ras, N-ras.

Important note: Expression of "ras" genes has been studied in both head and neck and oral cancer. Amplification and mutation of ras occur and frequently in southern Asia where malignancy accounts for 40% of all tumors; in contrast, ras mutations are very rare in the Western world.

3. *Gene transcription*: These genes make up a portion of transcription factor AP1 that binds to specific DNA sequences and enhances transcription. Examples include "fas" and "Jun".

4. *Apoptosis regulators*: The other group of proto-oncogenes are programmed cell death regulators. Examples include Bcl-1, Bcl-2.

Tumor Suppressor Genes

Tumor suppressor genes slow down the cell division and also encode proteins that may counteract the effect of proto-oncogenes. In normal cells, these genes modulate growth-promoting signals, transcription, DNA repair, and replication.

Deletion or mutational loss of function of tumor suppressor genes also contributes to tumorigenesis.

Among 30 tumor suppressor genes identified, the most important are p53 and Rb (retinoblastoma); p53 genes control:

1. Cell division
2. DNA repair
3. Apoptosis

This is a single gene copy located on the short arm of chromosome 17. The gene encodes a nuclear phosphoprotein that functions as a trans-activating transcriptional regulator that controls the expression of a set of genes important in regulation of cell cycle and in triggering apoptosis after certain types of genomic damage.

Functions of p53 genesa are as follows:

1. It binds to DNA and acts as a one of the master switches of transcription factors regulating gene activity.
2. It modulates transcription of p21 gene products which in turn inhibit progression of cell cycle.
3. It also increases the level of "fas", "bcl-1" gene that play important role in apoptosis.

Mechanism of Normal Apoptotic Pathway

Normal cells have very low p53 gene levels but whenever there is damage of DNA, level p53 rises dramatically.

If DNA damage is mild to moderate, the level of p53 increases which switches rise in p21 level. P21 is a cyclin-dependent kinase inhibitor (CDK inhibitor) that induces cell arrest in the G1 phase and transition arrest in the S phase. It further stops the cycle of cell progression until DNA repair occurs.

If this damage is severe, repair of DNA is not completed and the cell enters the apoptotic pathway and there is further increase in p53 gene and the cell dies.

Any alterations in p53 genes cause cells to grow out of control without programmed death, which leads to cancer. These alterations possibly involve at least four different molecular mechanisms. They are

1. p53 mutations
2. Deletion of wild type of alleles
3. Increased dosage of mutant gene
4. p53 gene amplification

The p53 mutation is claimed to be the most common genetic alteration associated with human cancer. More than 1000 p53 mutations have been identified in human neoplasms. The majority of mutations are found in the central 200 amino acid portion of the protein. However, all p53 mutations in cancer are not mutant. The normal p53 protein has a short half-life (20–30 min) and is not detected by immunohisto-chemistry, whereas the mutant form is stabilized and readily detected.

The overall percentage of p53 tumors in head and neck squamous cell carcinomas reported in the literature is 37%. Smoking is also shown to be inducer of p53 mutations in normal mucosa.

Other oncogenes are Rb (retinoblastoma), Bcl-2, etc.

Molecular Biomarkers of Cancer

Tumor markers are biochemical or biologic substances that are produced by tumors cells. They are then secreted into the urine, blood, and other body tissues or body fluids of patients with certain types of cancer in higher amounts than normal. A tumor marker might be produced by a primary tumor itself or can also be produced by the body's response to the presence of cancerous or noncancerous conditions.

Based on the ideology that primary tumor may harbor a distinct molecular biological information on the metastatic potential of the primary tumor, biomarkers have been extensively studied. Biomarkers not only aid in diagnosis but also determine the prognosis.

- These markers can be measured quantitatively or qualitatively by chemical, immunological, or molecular biological methods.
- Tumor markers can be estimated in the blood or in the tissues.
- Tumor markers can be directly identified within cells and tissues.
- Along with other diagnostic tests and measurement of tumor markers levels, it can be more useful in the diagnosis and detection of certain type of cancers.

Specimen Collection

- Tumor marker tests require 5–10 mL of a patient's blood. A tourniquet is tied on the elbow region of the patient's upper arm, the vein is identified and a needle is inserted. A vacuum in the middle draws the blood through the needle into an attached tube.
- Collection of the blood sample hardly takes a few minutes and results are available within a few days.

Method of Detection from Blood and Urine Samples

- Tumor marker tests usually are done by combining a sample with a substance which contains antibodies to these tumor markers.
- These antibodies bind to the markers and a radioactive substance is then added, to measure the amount of bound marker and antibodies.
- From the abovementioned measurement, the amount of tumor marker is then calculated.

Classification

1. Markers of enhanced tumor growth:
   - Epithelial growth factor (EGF)
   - Epithelial growth factor receptors (EGFR)
   - Cyclins
   - Proliferation cell nuclear antigen (PCNA)
   - Ki67

- Bcl-2, BAG-1
- Heat shock proteins

2. Markers of tumor suppression and antitumor response:
   - Retinoblastoma protein (Rb)
   - Cyclic-dependent kinase inhibitors
   - P53
   - Fas/fasl
   - Dendritic cells

3. Angiogenesis:
   - Vascular endothelial growth factor (VEGF)
   - Vascular endothelial growth factor receptor (VEGF-R)
   - Platelet-derived endothelial growth factor (PD-EGF)

4. Markers of tumor invasion and metastatic potential:
   - Matrix metalloproteins (MMP)
   - Cathepsins
   - Integrins
   - Cadherins
   - Desmoplakin
   - Ets-1

Clinical Applications of Tumor Markers

- *Screen*: Used to screen in those patients with a very strong family history of a particular cancer.
- In the case of genetic biomarkers, they can also be used to predict the risk of cancer in family members. Prostate-specific antigen (PSA) testing for prostate cancer is an example.
- *Help to diagnose*: In a patient who has clinical symptoms of cancer, tumor markers may be helpful to identify the etiology of the cancer, like CA-125 for ovarian cancer, and may also help to differentiate it from other various conditions/cancers.
- *Stage*: If a patient does have cancer, elevation of tumor marker elevations can be used to predict to determine the extent the cancer has spread into other body tissues and organs.
- *Determine prognosis*: Some tumor markers are often used by clinicians, which help to predict to determine how aggressive a cancer is likely to behave.
- *Guide treatment*: Some tumor markers, like Her2/neu, will give clinicians information about which modality treatments their patients might respond to.
- *Monitor treatment*: Tumor markers can also be used to observe the response of treatment, especially in locally advanced and metastatic cancers. If there is a drop in marker level, the tumor is responding; if the marker level stays elevated, alterations in management are needed.
- *Determine recurrence*: Presently, one of the major uses for tumor markers is to observe/monitor for recurrence of cancer. If there is elevation of tumor marker before treatment, low after treatment, and then again gradually begin to elevate over time, it is likely believed that there is a tumor recurrence. If it still remains elevated after surgery, the likelihood is that the tumor was incompletely resected.

Limitations of Tumor Markers

- False elevation of tumor marker may also be seen in nonneoplastic conditions as most of the tumor markers are composed of proteins and are over expressed not only by cancerous cells but it is expressed also by normal body tissues, e.g. CA-125 tumor marker that is elevated in epithelial ovarian cancer.

- Also many markers exhibit epitopes that cross-react with products of normal tissues, which might lead to errors in their quantitative estimation.
- Most the tumor markers do not cause allergy specific to a particular one type of cancer; the level of a tumor marker can be elevated in every by more than one type of cancer.
- In every person, tumor marker levels are not elevated with cancer especially in patients with the early stage of disease.
- No other simple diagnostic tests are available yet which provide sufficient sensitivity and specificity in detecting the presence of a cancerous cell. The field of tumor markers is still expanding with many updated new markers added either in clinical use or under active evaluation.

Emerging Trends in Molecular Biology

- Molecular biology is the most interesting trend that is emerging in this area to carefully understand the biological behavior of tumor.
- Another interesting trend presently being investigated is the use of the polymerase chain reaction (PCR) to check whether the surgical margins that were obtained during the time of surgery are histopathologically tumor free or contain a small amount of tumor cells that are histologically undetectable.
- Specifically, the utilization of PCR to detect specific gene mutations is important to determine if the prognosis and clinical outcome is affected by the presence of submicroscopic tumor cells.
- The recent advancement of in situ PCR might allow the amplification of both RNA and DNA directly in tissue section; this method must be extremely useful in the near future to localize the tumor cells that contain altered oncogenes or tumor suppressor genes.
- Molecular probes could also be used to help in early detection of second malignancies.

Recommendations

- Never depend on the results of one diagnostic test.
- When ordering several tests, make certain to order every test from the same diagnostic laboratory using the same assay kit.
- Always be certain that the selected tumor marker used for monitoring recurrence was seen elevated in the patient prior to surgery.
- Consider the half-life of the tumor marker when interpreting test results.
- Metabolization of the tumor marker from blood circulation must always be considered.
- We must consider ordering multiple markers to improve both specificity and the sensitivity for diagnosis.
- It is important to be aware of the presence of ectopic tumor markers.

Molecular Biomarkers in Oral Squamous Cell Carcinomas

Luo et al.[1] evaluated the importance of chemosensitivity and osteopontin (OPN) in locally advanced oral squamous cell carcinomas (OSCCs). They have studied 121 patients and validated the role of OPN in cell proliferation. They have put forward that the percentage of proliferation was relatively increased in matricellular OPN in a dose-dependent manner in SAS cells. The result of this study states that the most important role of OPN is to enhance the growth of OSCC cells. The authors have concluded that OPN-mediated cisplatin resistance often contributes to a poorer clinical outcome and altered local wound healing in patients with locally advanced inoperable OSCC managed with cisplatin-based chemoradiation.

Taoudi Benchekroun et al.[2] performed a retrospective study in which they investigated oral premalignant lesions (OPLs). The authors in there study indicated that it is common to find an increased *EGFR* gene copy number. The authors also put forward that an increased number of *EGFR* gene copies in

OPLs is a precursor to *EGFR* gene amplification in HNSCC. It is the most important oncogenesis-driving effector in oral oncogenesis thereby reducing the possibility of successful healing of the tissues at the surgical site.

Jung et al.[3] studied OSCCs in which they identified deregulated miRNAs and further focused on specific miRNAs that were found to be related to patient survival. Authors concluded that expression of miRNA profiling provided more apt information when OSCC were subcategorized on the basis of clinicopathological criteria. This study highlighted that different clinicopathological features and miRNA expression profiles can be used as specific hallmark for individual subtypes of oral tumors which has different final prognoses and good healing.

Minakawa et al.[4] thought that kinesin family member 4 (KIF4A) is majorly involved in OSCC pathogenesis by the activation of the spindle assembly checkpoint (SAC). KIF4A is overexpressed frequently in OSCC, and it suggests interference in the function of the spindle checkpoint proteins such as BUB1, MAD2, and CDC20. The authors reported that KIF4A expression is likely to be a key regulator of carcinogenesis progression in OSCCs. Su et al. studied how the DEPDC1B (defined like guanine nucleotide exchange factor) induced both cell migration in a cultured embryonic fibroblast cell line. The authors concluded that samples of oral cancer are overexpressed with DEPDC1B proteins, when compared with adjacent tissues that are normal, and so DEPDC1B plays a key role in the development of oral cancer.

Cao et al.[5] studied the role and importance of the transcriptional repressor called Enhancer of Zeste Homolog 2 (EZH2) in oral carcinogenesis and its clinical implication as a risk predictor of OSCC. The study showed that how, at 5 years after diagnosis, 80% of these patients expressed strong EZH2-developed OSCCs.

Saintigny et al.[6] considered deltaNp63 as a homolog of the p53 tumor suppressor that is most frequently amplified and overexpressed not only in OSCC but also in HNSCC.

REFERENCES

1. Luo S-D, Chen Y-J, Liu C-T et al. Osteopontin involves cisplatin resistance and poor prognosis in oral squamous cell carcinoma. *BioMed Research International*. 2015;2015:13.
2. Taoudi Benchekroun M, Saintigny P, Thomas SM et al. Epidermal growth factor receptor expression and gene copy number in the risk of oral cancer. *Cancer Prevention Research*. 2010;3(7):800–809.
3. Jung HM, Phillips BL, Patel RS et al. Keratinization-associated miR-7 and miR-21 regulate tumor suppressor reversion-inducing cysteine-rich protein with kazal motifs (RECK) in oral cancer. *Journal of Biological Chemistry*. 2012;287(35):29261–72.
4. Minakawa Y, Kasamatsu A, Koike H. et al. Kinesin family member 4A: a potential predictor for progression of human oral cancer. *PLoS One*. 2013;8(12).
5. Cao W, Younis RH, Li J et al. EZH2 promotes malignant phenotypes and is a predictor of oral cancer development in patients with oral leukoplakia. *Cancer Prevention Research*. 2011;4(11):1816–24.
6. Saintigny P, Zhang L, Fan YH et al. Gene expression profiling predicts the development of oral cancer. *Cancer Prevention Research*. 2011;4(2):218–29.

3

TNM Staging and Grading

History and Evolution of TNM Staging

- *1929*: League of Nations Health Organization
- *1953*: International Commission of Stage Grouping and Presentation of Results of the International Union against Cancer (UICC)
- *1954*: UICC TNM Committee (includes AJCC)
- *1976*: AJCC National Cancer Conference on Classification and Staging
- *1977*: AJCC Cancer Staging Manual (1st Edition)
- *1990*: Commission on Cancer mandates use of AJCC-TNM Staging System for all approved hospitals
- *2018*: Eighth edition of AJCC-UICC Staging System[1]

Philosophy

Cancers of the same anatomic site and histology share almost similar patterns of growth and prognostics outcomes. As the size of the primary tumor (T) increases, regional lymph node involvement (N) and/or distant metastases (M) become more likely[2].

- *TNM records the three significant events in the life history of a cancer patient*:
  - Local tumor growth (T)
  - Spread to regional lymph nodes (N)
  - Distant metastasis (M)
- *Histopathologic type*:
  - Qualitative assessment of categorization according to the cell type that a tumor most closely resembles
- *Histopathologic grade* (Broder's):
  - Qualitative assessment of the extent to which a tumor resembles the normal tissue at that site
    - *GX*: Grade cannot be assessed
    - *G1*: Well-differentiated carcinoma
    - *G2*: Moderately differentiated carcinoma
    - *G3*: Poorly differentiated carcinoma
- *Multiple simultaneous tumors*:
  - Classification and staging is based on the tumor that has the highest T category
  - Simultaneous bilateral cancers in paired organs are staged separately
- *Unknown primary*:
  - Staging can be based on clinical suspicion of the primary origin

DOI: 10.1201/9780367822019-3

Important notes:

- *Not all tumors behave in the same "TNM" fashion*
  - For example, lymphomas and Hodgkin's disease
  - Sarcomas (where the tumor size and histology are very important)

(For these and others, individualized staging systems are designed)

- *There is no reliable staging system for primary CNS cancers*
- *Pediatric tumors are outside the scope of this staging system*

Philosophy of Changes to TNM Staging

1. The introduction of new modalities with advanced technologies may require a modification of the classification system and staging systems.
2. However, there must be recognition of the kinetics of change in staging systems.
3. TNM staging has changes that may alter the treatment and outcome of the patient.
4. There may be changes that make it difficult to compare the outcomes of current therapy with those of previous treatment.

Therefore, changes must be undertaken with caution. Only factors validated in multiple large studies utilizing valid measures of cancer survival analysis have been incorporated into the staging system.

Advantages for Staging of Cancer

- Used to evaluate and compare groups of patients.
- Accurate clinical examination and histopathologic classification of malignant tumors may help to plan its objectives.
- Helps to select primary and adjuvant modality of treatments.
- Helps predict patient's prognosis.
- Assists in the evaluation of treatment results/outcomes.
- Facilitates the exchange of communication of information among various treatment centers/clinicians.
- Contributes to continuing investigation/management of human cancers.

TNM System

- *TNM system*: This is the expression of anatomic extent of the tumor which is based on three primary components for assessment:
  - *T*: Anatomic extent of primary tumor
  - *N*: The absence or presence and extent of regional lymph node metastasis
  - *M*: The absence or presence of distant metastasis
- The use of numerical subsets of TNM components indicates the progressive extent of the disease:
  - TX, T0, T1, T2, T3, T4
  - NX, N0, N1, N2, N3
  - MX, M0, M1

Classification for TNM Staging

- There are four classifications as described for each site:
  - Clinical classification (cTNM)
  - Pathological classification (pTNM)
  - Retreatment classification (rTNM)
  - Autopsy classification (aTNM)

Clinical Classification: cTNM

- Classification is assigned prior to any cancer-directed treatment
- It is based on physical examination/clinical examination, imaging, endoscopy, and biopsy
- It is used for selecting and evaluating primary mode of management

Pathological Classification: pTNM

- *Supplemented or modified*: Additional evidence acquired during and from surgery
- *Additional precise data*: Estimates prognosis and calculates the end results of the patient
- *pT*: Resection of the primary tumor with several other partial removals
- *pN*: Removes sufficient number of lymph nodes

Retreatment Classification: rTNM

- When further management is planned for a tumor that recurs after disease-free intervals
- All information at the time of retreatment—determines the stage of the recurrent tumor (rTNM)

Autopsy Classification: aTNM

- Postmortem classification of tumor performed after the death of a patient
- Staging is done with all the pathological information—at the time of death

Staging into Groups

- After clinical and pathological assessment of the primary tumor, grouping into stages is done
- *Carcinoma* in *situ (CIS)*: Exception to stage group guidelines. Only biopsy-proven squamous cell carcinoma is grouped in TNM staging
- *pTis, cN0, cM0*: Clinical stage group 0

For multiple tumors:

- *Multiple tumors in one region/organ*: Highest T category is selected
- Multiplicity or number of tumors are indicated in brackets (T2[m], T2[5])
- *In thyroid gland*: Multiplicity is criterion of T classification
- *For unknown primary tumors*: Staging is only based on clinical suspicion of primary origin

TNM staging shall be discussed in the next individual chapters based on anatomical areas.

REFERENCES

1. Shah JP, Montero PH. New AJCC/UICC staging system for head and neck, and thyroid cancer. *Revista Médica Clínica Las Condes*. 2018 Jul 1;29(4):397–404.
2. Edge SB, Compton CC. The American Joint Committee on Cancer: The 7th edition of the AJCC Cancer Staging Manual and the Future of TNM. *Annals of Surgical Oncology*. 2010 Jun 1;17(6):1471–1474.

4

Lymphatic System and Lymph Nodes

This system is described after the other parts of vascular system are already known. The reason for this delay is their delicate, transparent appearance and complex system.

Embryology

- *Lymph sacs*: These appear between 2nd and 6th weeks of intrauterine life.
- *7th week*: Jugular channel spreads to connect with subclavian lymph sacs.
- *9th week*: Thoracic duct is a continuous channel draining into internal jugular vein and subclavian vein junction.
- *12th week*: All the processes of lymph sac formation are complete.
- *5th month*: Valves begin to start developing.

What Is Lymph?

- Lymph is defined as a transudative fluid that flows from the interstitium to enter the lymphatic capillaries. Interstitial fluid is formed because it is permeable to the arterial end of the capillaries.
  - *Lymph composition*: Lyumph is composed of 96% water and 4% solids (lipids, carbohydrates, proteins, electrolytes, and blood cells chiefly lymphocytes).

Functions of Lymph

- It returns the lost interstitial fluid back to the vascular system at a rate of 100–120 ml/h.
- It returns the plasma proteins that are lost back to the vascular system.
- It carries absorbed substances/nutrients (e.g. fat chylomicrons) from GI tract.
- Defense function: It helps to remove bacteria, toxins, and foreign bodies from the tissues.

Lymphatic System

Lymphatic system consists of:

- Lymphatic capillaries
- Lymphatic vessels
- Lymph nodes

Lymphatic Capillaries

Lymphatic capillaries are closed microscopic ended vessels that are lined by a thin flat endothelial cell in a single layer that is situated in tissue spaces next to blood capillaries and are larger in diameter than

DOI: 10.1201/9780367822019-4

blood capillaries. They are very permeable and collect tissue fluid and proteins. Lymphatic capillaries merge together to form larger group of lymph vessels.

Lymphatic Vessels

These vessels are similar to the venous system but often have more valves with thinner walls. The ends of these endothelial cells overlap with each other to act as one-way valves that allow the interstitial fluid to flow in one direction from inside but not outside. The tissue that surrounds them is attached by anchoring filaments. There is no pump mechanism for lymph vessels. The movement of the lymph occurs by constriction of vessels, skeletal muscle pump, and respiratory pump. Lymph trunks are formed by unity of lymphatic vessels.

Lymph Trunks

Lymph trunks are formed by uniting large tubes of lymphatic vessels that empty their lymph into these lymphatic ducts.

Lymph Ducts

The following two conducting ducts drain the lymphatic ducts:

- The thoracic duct also called left lymphatic duct
- The right lymphatic duct

Lymph fluid from these ducts enters the bloodstream via the left and right subclavian veins, respectively.

Lymph Nodes

Lymph nodes are oval and bean-shaped glands. Lymphatic tissues are collective masses that help as defense mechanisms and the formation of white blood cells (WBCs). Lymph nodes are located along the entire length of lymphatic vessels and are also scattered usually in clusters throughout the body.

Lymph nodes are usually covered by a capsule that has trabeculae that are capsular extensions. They are partitions within a node. There are reticular fibers that fibroblasts in the capsule that help to form the framework of a lymph node. Lymph nodes have two main parts, cortex and medulla.

Functions of Lymph Nodes

- As lymph passes through these nodes, microorganisms such as bacteria and other foreign materials trap these by their reticular fibers within a node. These microorganisms are then phagocytized by macrophages.
- Antibodies are produced by plasma cells in response to antigens in the lymph.
- The subclavian vein eventually receives the return of these antibodies, lymphocytes, and monocytes to the blood.

The major groups of lymph nodes are as follows:

- Cervical lymph nodes
- Axillary lymph nodes
- Mediastinal lymph nodes
- Inguinal lymph nodes
- Mesenteric lymph nodes
- Retroperitoneal lymph nodes

Head and Neck Lymphatics[1]

Conventionally, lymphatics of the head and neck are divided into three systems

- Waldeyer's internal ring
- Superficial lymph node system, also called Waldeyer's external ring
- Deep lymph node system (cervical lymph nodes proper)

Waldeyer's Internal Ring

Waldeyer's internal ring refers to a collection of lymphoid tissue in a circular form similar to a ring within the pharynx at the skull base. It forms a ring that includes adenoids, palatine tonsils, tubal and lingual tonsils and aggregates on the posterior pharyngeal wall.

Superficial Nodal System (Also Called "Waldeyer's External Ring")

These drain the superficial tissues of the head and neck region and consist of two circles of nodes, one in the head and the other in the neck.

- *In head*: These nodes, also known as occipital, postauricular, parotid or preauricular, buccal, and facial nodes, are situated around the base of skull.
- *In neck*: Here, these can be classified into submental, submandibular, and anterior cervical nodes.

Deep Lymph Nodal System

Deeper fascial tissues of the head and neck drain either directly through the superficial system or into the deep cervical nodes. They consist of:

1. Junctional nodes
2. Internal jugular nodes
3. Spinal accessory nodes
4. Supraclavicular nodes
5. Nuchal nodes
6. Deep medial visceral nodes

Important note: Tumor dissemination via regional lymphatics to lymph node groups occurs in a sequential and predictable fashion—Dr. Jatin P Shah.

Classification of Lymph Nodes in the Neck[2]

Occipital lymph nodes: These lie on the upper end of the trapezius muscle and on the fascia at the apex of the posterior triangle. They usually drain the occipital portion of the scalp and the upper portion behind the neck to the upper deep cervical lymph nodes under cover of sterno-cleidomastoid muscle (SCM).

Retro auricular lymph nodes: These are also called mastoid nodes and lie on the superior portion of the SCM and are posterior to the auricle. These lymph nodes drain the posterior half of the side of the head and the posterior surface of the auricle to deep nodes under the SCM.

Parotid lymph nodes: These are several small nodes scattered through out the parotid gland.

The superficial nodes drain the area from a vertical line through the auricle forward to an oblique line joining the angle of mandible to the medial angle of the eye, including most of the auricle and the external acoustic meatus.

Deeper nodes drain the temporal and infratemporal fossa, the middle ear auditory tube, and upper molar teeth and gingiva—they pass to either nodes in the external jugular vein (EJV) or to the upper deep cervical nodes.

> *Submandibular lymph nodes*: These nodes surround the submandibular gland mainly under the lower border of the mandible, they receive superficial lymph dressing from the area below the line joining the medial angle of the eye and the angle of the mandible.

Deeper lymph vessels drain the sublingual and submandibular salivary glands, the lateral border of the tongue, posterior part of the floor of the mouth, most of the teeth and gingiva, also part of the palate and the anterior walls of the nasal cavity.

Its efferent passes to deep cervical nodes under the SCM. Some small lymph nodes lie along the course of facial veins, one of these lie at the anterior border of masseter called the mandibular node or a node of starr. It drains the cheeks and lateral parts of the lips to the submandibular nodes.

> *Submental lymph nodes*: These nodes lie on the fascia covering the mylohyoid muscle, between the two anterior bellies of digastric muscle. They drain the lymph from wedge-shaped zone that includes the incisor teeth and their gingiva. The anterior part of the floor of the mouth ultimately drains into deep cervical nodes, some vessels passing with the anterior jugular vein drain to the lower group.

> *Retropharyngeal lymph nodes*: A few lymph nodes lie on the fascia of the posterior wall of the upper pharynx and at the level of the mastoid process. These lymph nodes drain from the oral and nasal parts of the pharynx, paranasal sinuses, palate, nose, auditory tube, and middle ear. These nodes drain postero-inferiorly to nodes in the posterior triangle.

Cervical Lymph Nodes

> *Superficial cervical nodes*: Three or four superficial nodes lie along the course of the EJV; they drain the parotid nodes and the adjoining skin either across the SCM to deep nodes in the carotid triangle or with the vein to deep nodes at the root of the neck. A few other small nodes on the anterior jugular vein drain surrounding skin and the muscles along the vein to the lower deep cervical lymph nodes.

> *Anterior cervical lymph nodes*: A few small nodes lie on the front and lateral sides of trachea most commonly besides the recurrent laryngeal nerves (RLNs). They are continuous below the tracheobronchial nodes in the thorax. They drain the lymph from the larynx, trachea, and thyroid gland to the lower deep cervical nodes.

Deep Cervical Lymph Nodes

Deep cervical lymph nodes form a broad strip of nodes in carotid sheath, from the digastric to the root of the neck mostly under cover of the SCM.

Two of the nodes are particularly large:

- Jugulodigastric group
- Jugulo-omohyoid group

The deep cervical nodes are linked by afferent and efferent vessels and receive lymph from all the other groups, their final efferent pathway for all the lymph nodes of the head and neck is the jugular lymph trunk at the root of the neck.

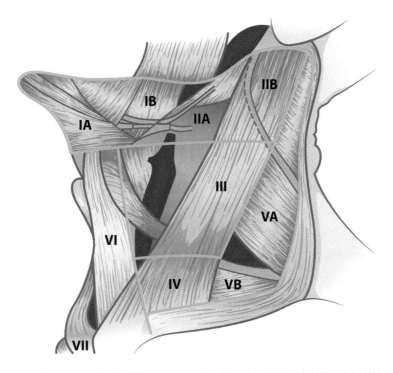

FIGURE 4.1   Cervical lymph nodal levels. This trunk enters the "thoracic duct" on the left and the IJV on the right.

LYMPH node levels (Figure 4.1):

- LEVEL I
  - IA—Submental nodes
  - IB—Submandibular nodes
- LEVEL II=> Upper jugular nodes
  - IIA—Anterior to SAN (Spinal accessory nerve)
  - IIB—Posterior to SAN
- LEVEL III => Mid jugular
- LEVEL IV =>Lower jugular nodes
  - IVA—Behind sternal end of SCM
  - IVB—Behind clavicular end of SCM
- LEVEL V => Anterior compartment

Palpation of Cervical Lymph Nodes

A systematic examination should be carried out to palpate all lymph nodal groups in the neck. It can be started from below the neck to the supraclavicular group and then moving upward palpating the lymph nodes in the posterior triangle, then jugulo-omohyoid group, after that the jugulodigastric, submandibular, submental, preauricular, and occipital groups.

The swelling in the neck is palpated from behind the patient, while patient is sitting, patient's head is passively flexed with one hand on their head and the other hand is used for palpating the swelling.

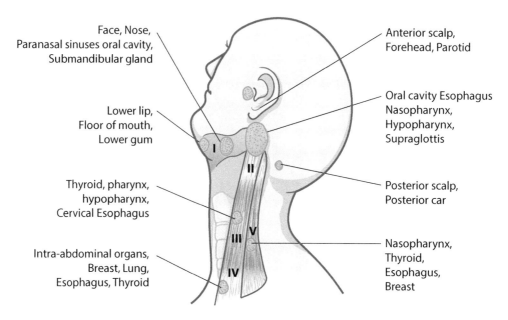

FIGURE 4.2   Pattern of Lymphatic drainage.

- **Oral cavity—I, II, III levels**
- **Oropharynx}**
- **Hypopharynx}   - II, III, IV**
- **Larynx   }**
- **Posterior scalp}**
- **Midline posterior neck} - V**
- **Nuchal skin}**
- **Thyroid   }**
- **Cervical trachea}   - VI**
- **Cervical esophagus}**

Submandibular lymph node: Stand behind the patient and flexing the neck toward the side of examination, nodes can be viewed in the submandibular region around the submandibular gland on the medial aspect of lower border of body mandible. If required, it can be palpated bimanually, from intraorally and extraorally simultaneously.

Submental lymph nodes: In the submental triangle between the anterior bellies of the digastric, can also be palpated bimanually.

TABLE 4.1

Distribution of Metastasis in Various Nodal Sites

Level of Nodes	Distribution (%)
Jugulodigastric (Level II)	71
Mid jugular (Level III)	72
Supraclavicular (Level IV)	18
Submandibular (Level IB)	12
Posterior triangle(Level V)	12
Submental (IA)	8

Superficial cervical group: Neck is flexed toward the side of examination, and the SCM in a relaxed position; the SCM is held in between the thumb and other fingers and rolled downward between them from above.

Supraclavicular group: This is palpated just above the clavicle by relaxing the muscles over the area.

Inspection

Swellings identify and document the number, position, size, surface, etc.

Skin over the swelling:

- *Acute*: Inflamed with redness, edema, and brawny induration
- *Chronic*: Normal

Pressure effects are dyspnea, congestion, etc.

Palpation is used for different sensations such as number, situation, local temperature, tenderness, and surface margin.

Consistency: Palpated with palmar aspect of three fingers against the swelling, slight pressure is maintained to know the consistency.

- *Soft*: Acute lymphadenitis
- *Elastic or rubbery*: Hodgkin's disease
- *Firm discrete and snotty*: Syphilis
- *Stony hard*: Secondary CA
- *Variable*: Soft to firm to hard depending on the rate of growth—lymphosarcoma

Matted lymph nodes or not—periadenitis and fusion of adjoining nodes—TB, acute lymphadenitis, secondary CA, etc.

Fixity to the surrounding structures—primary malignant growth of lymph nodes, lymph sarcoma, reticulosarcoma, histosarcoma, or secondary CA—is often fixed.

Investigations

- Biopsy
- *Radiological examination*: To check whether calcified TB nodes, tomography and also to check for mediastinal nodes
- Lymphangiography
- *Mediastinal scanning*: Ga67
- *Laparotomy*: Hodgkin's disease
- *MRI*: Functional MRI

Management

Management aspects vary according to the etiology of the lymph node enlargement.

- *Acute and chronic enlargement*: It may regress once the focus of infection is treated.
- *Granulomatous enlargement*: It may regress once the systemic disease is treated. Sometime excision might be required.
- *Secondary CAs*: Surgical treatment or radiotherapy or (RTP+surgery+RTP) or chemotherapy alone or in combination.

Pan, Wei-Ren et al. performed a study to relocate lymphatic system draining from superficial tissues of the head and neck regions over 20 years in 18 halves from 9 fresh cadavers. They concluded that the lymph capillaries draining from the galea aponeurotica layers and the skin sequentially get collected into precollecting lymph vessels, then collecting lymphatics and then the first-tier/echelon lymph nodes. The diameter of these collecting vessels averages from 0.2 mm in with unusual structures called "lymphatic ampullae." There are different lymphatic pattern network between every patient and between the sides of the same patient. Similar relationships exist between the lymphatic and venous systems with a lymphati-covenous shunt in the occipital region. Sometimes lymphatics bypass the expected nodes to reach their first echelon sentinel nodes in the root of the neck and the lymphatics of the anterior neck lying above the platysma and coursing obliquely, horizontally and upward and toward the mandible[2].

REFERENCES

1. Watkinson J, Gilbert R. *Stell & Maran's textbook of head and neck surgery and oncology.* CRC Press; 2011 Dec 30.
2. Shah JP, Patel SG, Singh B. *Head and neck surgery and oncology.* Elsevier Health Sciences; 2012.
3. Pan WR, Suami H, Taylor GI. Lymphatic drainage of the superficial tissues of the head and neck: anatomical study and clinical implications. *Plastic and Reconstructive Surgery.* 2008 May 1;121(5):1614–24.

5

Imaging

Ultrasonography

USG is a simple and reliable, and a primary valuable imaging tool for metastatic lymph node evaluation in HNSCC patients. It is an economical and noninvasive diagnostic method. USG is a better modality than clinical palpation in detecting very small cervical metastatic nodes.

Computed Tomography Scan

Computed tomography (CT) scans give valuable information not only about the soft tissue status but also of soft tissue structures like organs, nerves and the brain and other exquisite detail of even the smallest bony structures like vertebrae. Paranasal sinus can be best studied by CT scans that also help in evaluating swelling, inflammation, and tumors (Figure 5.1).

Advantages

- A quick investigation, which is easily available, that gives exact details of useful anatomic information.
- It can be done with different sequences, which can effectively evaluate veins and arteries.
- It is excellent for showing bone anatomy.
- It may also be used to guide a placement of a needle for performing biopsies.

Disadvantages

- CT scan can expose patients to radiation. A CT scan has benefits that far outweigh any risks from radiation exposure when used correctly. In certain situations, a magnetic resonance imaging (MRI) scan could be used an alternative to a CT scan.
- Images can be degraded and deformed with movement and dental fillings/prosthesis.
- It only shows late changes associated with an invasion of nerves such as the destruction of foramen as the nerve enters the skull.

Magnetic Resonance Imaging

An MRI scan can be critical to planning the surgery, radiation therapy or managing any other disorders of the head and neck area. Although it is not as precise and accurate in evaluating bony structures as CT scan but MRI always gives superior detail of soft tissue structures like nerves, the spinal cord and the brain. When considering tumors, MRI is better when compared to CT in assessing or describing these soft tissue masses. MRIs are best used to monitor/locate cranial nerve injuries and disorders, including

---

DOI: 10.1201/9780367822019-5

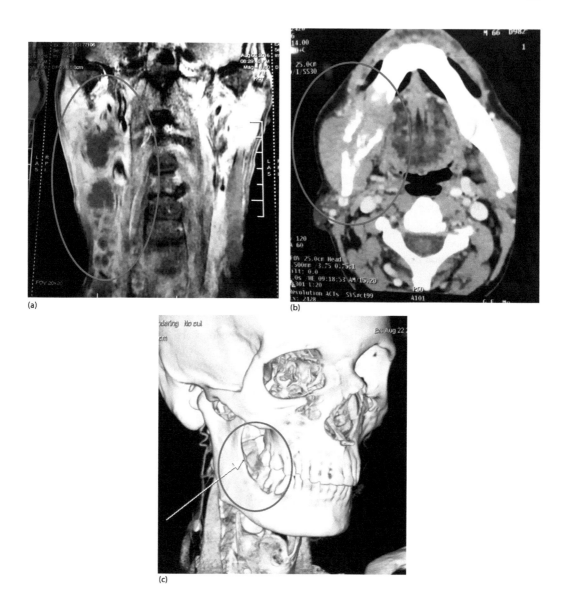

FIGURE 5.1   (a) This is coronal section of a CT scan of a carcinoma patient showing necrotic lymph nodes on the right side. (b) This axial section of a CT scan shows a huge lower alveolus lesion on the right side destructing both the cortical plates. (c) This is a three-dimensional reconstruction scan showing erosion of the buccal cortex at angle—ramus unit.

brain and spinal cord tumors and tissue abnormalities in persons with orbital or inner ear pathologies (Figure 5.2).

Advantages

- There is no radiation involved.
- Details of the soft tissues are fine and better than that of a CT scan.
- They show earlier pickup of nerves and the involvement of the skull base.

Disadvantages

- They take much longer than a CT scan and are more costly.
- Even a slight movement and dental prosthesis can degrade the images.

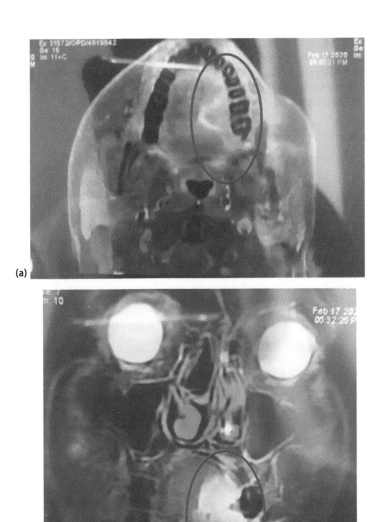

FIGURE 5.2 (a) Axial section of MRI scan showing a lesion of lateral border of the tongue on the left side extending to the anterior tip to the anterior tonsillar pillar. (b) Coronal section of MRI scan showing a lesion of the lateral border of the tongue on the left side involving the genioglossus and part of the mylohyoid muscle in the floor of mouth.

- Some people feel claustrophobic inside MRI machines.
- There can be huge banging noise inside the machine, which might be uncomfortable.

Zoran Rumboldt et al. performed a study and stated that MRI scans are the most preferred modality of investigation for study and clinical examination of sinonasal, nasopharyngeal and parotid gland tumors since it has excellent contrast resolution with less prominent motion artifacts and a very high frequency of evaluation of perineural spread. MRI scan is the appropriate mode of investigation to define the anatomical extent of intracranial and intraorbital extension of malignant tumors. CT scans are primarily used to image tumors of oral cavity and oropharynx, larynx and hypopharynx, where breathing and swallowing does not give any motion artifacts. MRI scan is also the primary modality of choice for lesions that are confined and subjected to the oral cavity, especially the oral tongue and other anatomical sites of oral cavity because it has superior image quality detection of the spread of tumor into the bone marrow. There is no clear advantage of MRI or CT scan for the evaluation of lymph nodal disease. Positron emission tomography (PET) is very sensitive for metastatic lymph nodes that are metastatic and at least 8 mm in diameter. It is a technique of choice in doubtful cases.

Imaging in Distant Metastasis

Distant metastasis is typically rare at initial presentation and depends considerably depends on the anatomic location of the primary tumor as well as initial T and N stages of the tumor. Pulmonary metastasis is the most common in head and neck cancers while liver, bone, mediastinal and skin metastasis are the other less common sites. Preoperative imaging of chest is done in every case as part of preanesthetic consent as well as to find any lung metastasis. Contrast CT of the chest is eventually done in those cancer patients with stage IV disease with a high risk for pulmonary metastasis where X-ray of the chest may be doubtful. With the introduction of PET-CT scan imaging, it may often be one among the imaging modality considered for initial staging. It also helps in the identification of associated second primary cancers. However, there must be more studies to prove the cost-effectiveness of PET-CT scan when compared with cross-sectional imaging for the initial staging of these tumors.

Role of Fusion Imaging: PET-CT Scan

^{18}F-fluorodeoxy-D-glucose PET-CT (^{18}F-FDG PET-CT) has become an important and valuable diagnostic tool for the radiological evaluation and prognostication of HNSCC. It is also applied in various clinical stages, that is, from pretreatment staging to radiation therapy planning and is also used in the assessment of post neoadjuvant treatment response assessment. Although ^{18}F-FDG is a PET tracer that is most commonly used for oncologic purposes, there are certain limitations in use in HNSCCs due to its complex anatomy and smaller size of the anatomical structures, as well as the physiological uptake of ^{18}F-FDG in normal organs having high mitotic activity that may influence image interpretation. ^{18}FDG uptake targets and reflects metabolism of glucose, which can also be observed in several normal human tissues with varied values of the normal uptake pattern, including brain, salivary glands, vocal cords, lymphoid tissue and brown fat, cervical muscles as well as in various benign tumors, such as common Warthin's tumor. Moreover, inflammatory processes occur in patients after the surgery or radiotherapy. False positive PET results are a frequent reason since there is increased ^{18}F-FDG uptake due to activated inflammatory cells. Finally, artifacts associated with the patient movement of the patient or metallic dental prostheses may further limit the interpretation of PET images, thus requiring non-attenuation corrected PET data evaluation. There are PET-CT scanners that allow high and quick resolution of the image, which can correlate anatomical location with functional information. The recent technological advancement of whole-body PET-MRI in oncologic practice offers new opportunities for integrated functional-anatomic imaging[1].

The clinical advantage and role of FDG PET-CT for the detection of involvement of lymph nodes and recurrence in patients with head and neck cancer is very well documented. It has been found to be the gold standard for imaging workups within the evaluation with HNSCC patients. FDG PET is additionally found to be more accurate and definite when compared to CT/MRI imaging in oral cavity cancer. There are potential clinical applications that include pretreatment staging, treatment monitoring and evaluation of the previously treated patients. The current oncological practice is not in favor of using PET-CT for staging of all newly diagnosed SCCs. However, PET scan can detect metastatic cervical lymph nodes that can be occult clinically and may not be detected by conventional CT or MRI. It can also detect primary HNSCCs that have a dimension greater than 1 cm in size. PET-CT may be performed in squamous cell carcinoma to evaluate for possible occult distant metastases to the lungs, liver or bones.

The presence of pulmonary metastases in PET-CT upstages a patient from M0 to M1 and alters the management. Routine imaging workup for the patient with pulmonary SCC includes a conventional radiography or CT scan of the chest at most of the centers. Though incidence is only 10% for distant metastasis in HNSCC, sometimes the surgeon fails to evaluate the distant metastasis because of nonavailability of PET-CT scanning equipment or due to its financial cost that the patient may not be able to to afford. But appropriate steps must be taken based on the clinical symptoms of the patients, which must not be ignored by the surgeon and PET-CT scan must be done, which can change the entire treatment management of the patient (Figure 5.3)[2–4].

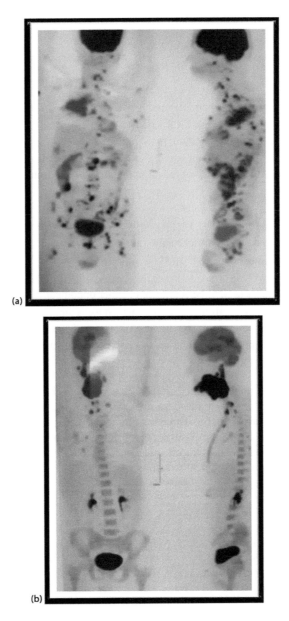

(a)

(b)

FIGURE 5.3 (a) FDG uptake with extensive metastasis to the vertebral column, bilateral supraclavicular and mediastinal nodes and other organs like the lung, liver, and long bones. (b) Increased FDG uptake in bilateral supraclavicular right pectoral and mediastinal nodes, increased metabolic activity of necrotic nodule in the superior segment of the right lower lobe of the lung.

Indications

1. Primary tumor identification
2. Nodal metastasis
3. Distant staging
4. Carcinoma of unknown primary
5. Treatment response assessment
6. Residual disease
7. Recurrent disease
8. Radiation planning
9. Post-therapy follow-up

Advantages

- The radioactive tracer decays soon after and hence PET scans have very little radiation.
- When PET scan is combined with a CT or MRI scan, a surgeon can combine anatomic and functional imaging techniques to obtain more precise and accurate information.
- In some cases, PET scans are much better and more reliable to distinguish cancer from other abnormalities related to the effects of radiation that might be present on an MRI or CT scan.

Disadvantages

- The results of PET scan imaging are less precise than anatomic studies such as CT scans and MRIs.
- It takes more time, and patient must remain totally still.
- PET scans are much more expensive and less available.
- The functional images alone do not delineate the specific organ or other structures that are hyper-metabolic. These images need to be combined together or compared with anatomic imaging.
- PET scans do not pick up small foci of tumors which use a significant amount of glucose. The tumor greater than 1 cm is easy to pick up for PET scanners
- The PET scan also lights up anatomic areas that are not necessarily cancer, which includes infected areas, since these cells also consume large amounts of glucose.

^{18}F-FDG PET-CT scan is predominantly used for staging, restaging and radiotherapy planning as well as for the assessment of treatment response in HNSCC patients, due to its superior accuracy over clinical examination and conventional techniques of imaging. The main limitations, especially in the posttreatment setting, are possibly false positive results due to inflammation and the inability to detect microscopic disease. In the future, new tracers other than ^{18}F-FDG, as well as PET-MRI imaging, will provide clear advantages in several clinical scenarios.

REFERENCES

1. Rumboldt Z, Gordon L, Bonsall R, Ackermann S. Imaging in head and neck cancer. *Current Treatment Options in Oncology*. 2006 Feb 1;7(1):23–34. https://link.springer.com/article/10.1007/s11864-006-0029-2#auth-1
2. Mohammad A, Bhargava A, Wadhwania A. Role of PET-CT scan in locally advanced head & neck cancer: a prospective study. *Journal of Head & Neck Physicians and Surgeons*. 2016 Jul 1;1(2):31.
3. Ryan WR, Fee Jr WE, Le QT, Pinto HA. Positron-emission tomography for surveillance of head and neck cancer. *Laryngoscope*. 2005 Apr;115(4):645–50.
4. Lowe VJ, Boyd JH, Dunphy FR, Kim H, Dunleavy T, Collins BT, Martin D, Stack Jr BC, Hollenbeak C, Fletcher JW. Surveillance for recurrent head and neck cancer using positron emission tomography. *Journal of Clinical Oncology*. 2000 Feb 1;18(3):651.

6

Sentinel Node Biopsies (SNBs)

Basis of Sentinel Lymph Nodes

- "It is the first lymph node to drain the lymph from a primary tumor of a specific anatomic site."
- It is based on a concept that a tumor will have a systematic nodal drainage basin, with a primary node.
- Seaman/Powers in 1955 proposed the first-echelon lymph node, a nodal basin with radioactive colloid gold.
- Gould in 1960 labeled the first-echelon node as the "sentinel node."
- Cabanas in 1977 identified specific a groin node in primary penile cancer.
- Morton in 1992 demonstrated intraoperative mapping in humans with melanoma using dye.

Roles of Sentinel Lymph Node Biopsies

- Potentially lessen morbidity of large surgical resection
- Guide treatment approaches (further neck dissection, radiation therapy, etc.)
- Facilitate further research of drainage patterns
- Help to find the prognosis of the patient
- Detect earlier stage "micrometastases"

Challenges

- High density of lymph nodes
- Close proximity to primary tumor
- Complex lymphatic pathways
- Optimization of localization and imaging essential for success

Sentinel Lymph Node Techniques

1. Dye peritumoral injection
2. Preoperative dynamic scintigraphy
   - Planar imaging
   - Single-photon emission CT (SPECT)/CT
3. Intraoperative static scintigraphy

DOI: 10.1201/9780367822019-6

Techniques

Dye Injection

- Injection of isosulfan blue dye submucously around tumor
- Nodes stain blue in 15–45 minutes after injection
- Exposure of nodal basin
- Removal of stained node

Limitations of Dye

- Invasiveness of broad exposure
- Dye spillage around tumor that leads to obscure margins
- 0.7–2% risk of anaphylaxis
- Skin tattooing
- Delay in dye washout

Radiolabeled Tracer

- Scintigraphy relies upon radioactive tracer
- Ideal particle size 5–10 nm—smaller particles may be taken into vascular system
- Gold, iodine, technetium have been used
- 99mTc attached to sulfur colloid or human albumin most commonly used tracer
- Investigation into other agents
  - Lymphoseek—dextran-based product, average size 5 nm
- Half-life is 6 hours
- Radioactivity detected 3–6 hours after injection
- Ideally surgery can be done the same day as injection

Lymphoscintigraphy

- Radiolabeled colloid injection around tumor periphery
- Gamma camera visualizes dynamic real-time flow to sentinel nodes
- Static images in anteroposterior/lateral views can be obtained
- Allows marking the site of the localized "hot spot" on the skin
- Need to keep patient in static position until marking is done

SPECT/CT Scintigraphy

- Use of CT scanners as opposed to planar imaging
- Combination with SPECT
- Better resolution of nodes adjacent to primary tumor where "shine through" obscures identification
- Better definition of nodes relative to anatomical landmarks
- Improved attenuation and scatter of gamma rays improves localization

Intraoperative Static Lymphoscintigraphy (ISL)

- Use of handheld gamma probe to identify node
- Nodes with peak readings are removed
- Any adjacent nodes with >10% activity are also removed

- Confirmation of excised nodes for positive activity
- Remaining bed should have less than 10% activity
- SLN ranked according to activity uptake ex vivo

Important Note—It is unpredictable due to:

1. Incidence is 5–10%
2. Predictive factors (review of 121 patients, 12 unsuccessful)
   a. Location, floor of mouth/anterior tongue
   b. T stage (higher stage more unsuccessful)
   c. Preoperative lymphoscintigraphy (LS) negative
3. "Shine through" from primary tumor can obscure identification
4. Tumor filling a node, distorting architecture, could redirect lymphatic flow
5. Suspicious nodes should be removed for that reason
6. Tumor size can directly compress draining lymphatics
7. Chemoradiation may alter drainage pathways

SPECT/CT Scan Used for Mapping SNBs

In addition to the described imaging procedure, SPECT can be used in a preoperative LS technique, which has advanced systems composed of a gamma camera and a CT scan that is fit on the same device has been recently introduced into clinical practice. SPECT and CT scans are acquired at the same clinical setting without even need for changing the patient's position and thus allowing for generation of apt and accurate fused images combining the functional data of SPECT scan and the anatomical data of the CT scan. Many studies from different institutions have reported many contradictory results on their clinical expertise with SPECT/CT scan for mapping of SLN in early oral squamous cell carcinoma[1,2].

Even-Sapir et al.[3] in 2000 performed a study that described the combination of data of the SPECT LS with a CT scan having a hybrid gamma camera and a low-dose CT scan system that allows SPECT and CT to be performed at the similar time without changing the position of the patient. The same author later introduced the use of hybrid SPECT/CT system with mapping of sentinel node of HNSCC, 3 years later.

Lopez et al.[4] studied 10 patients and stated that SPECT/CT scans shall become a important and useful tool for SNBs, which was later confirmed by Wagner et al.[5] in their study. They have found an additional lymph node probably lymph node of starr nearby the submandibular gland that was only been detected and identified by SPECT/CT scan. This lymph node has always been missed by conventional planar LS and the intraoperative gamma probe due to the scattering of the radioactive material from the primary tumor that hindered the location of the radiolabeled SLNs. The similar problem has been shown by several authors in the earlier period of radio-guided imaging and was thought be identified by introducing SPECT/CT scan.

Thomsen et al.[6] in their study found that those SLNs that were very close to the primary tumor were very difficult to detect and have oblique planar images and/or tomographic scans were added that would help to rectify this issue. Terada et al. also performed a pilot study on SPECT/CT and head and neck mucosal carcinomas and concluded that they were able to detect out all the SLNs with the help of fusion images and gamma probe was used to confirm its radioactivity without the adverse effect of overlapping radioactivity from the primary tumor site. Khafif et al.[7] performed a study in 22 patients with biopsy-proven OSCC and found an improved identification of the SLNs with SPECT/CT in 30% compared to planar imaging. Bilde et al. in their study included 34 stage I and II patients OSCC undergoing planar LS and SPECT/CT. He concluded that SPECT/CT demonstrated an extra SLN in 47% when compared to LS alone.

Therefore, SPECT/CT scan has a great benefit to detect or enhance more SLNs, which might harbor occult disease, when compared to traditional LS technique alone. Irrespective, with regard to the excellent and promising results achieved with LS and the intraoperative use of the gamma probe, SPECT/CT is not indispensable and feasible for successful SNBs.

REFERENCES

1. Shoaib T, Soutar DS, MacDonald DG, Camilleri IG, Dunaway DJ, Gray HW, McCurrach GM, Bessent RG, MacLeod TI, Robertson AG. The accuracy of head and neck carcinoma sentinel lymph node biopsy in the clinically N0 neck. *Cancer: Interdisciplinary International Journal of the American Cancer Society*. 2001 Jun 1;91(11):2077–83.
2. Thompson CF, John MS, Lawson G, Grogan T, Elashoff D, Mendelsohn AH. Diagnostic value of sentinel lymph node biopsy in head and neck cancer: a meta-analysis. *European Archives of Oto-Rhino-Laryngology*. 2013 Jul 1;270(7):2115–22.
3. Even-Sapir E, Lerman H, Lievshitz G, Khafif A, Fliss DM, Schwartz A, Gur E, Skornick Y, Schneebaum S. Lymphoscintigraphy for sentinel node mapping using a hybrid SPECT/CT system. *Journal of Nuclear Medicine*. 2003 Sep 1;44(9):1413–20.
4. Lopez R, Payoux P, Gantet P, Esquerré JP, Boutault F, Paoli JR. Multimodal image registration for localization of sentinel nodes in head and neck squamous cell carcinoma. *Journal of Oral and Maxillofacial Surgery*. 2004 Dec 1;62(12):1497–504.
5. Wagner A, Schicho K, Glaser C, Zettinig G, Yerit K, Lang S, Klug C, Leitha T. SPECT-CT for topographic mapping of sentinel lymph nodes prior to gamma probe-guided biopsy in head and neck squamous cell carcinoma. *Journal of Cranio-Maxillofacial Surgery*. 2004 Dec 1;32(6):343–9.
6. Thomsen JB, Sørensen JA, Grupe P, Krogdahl A. Sentinel lymph node biopsy in oral cancer: validation of technique and clinical implications of added oblique planar lymphoscintigraphy and/or tomography. *Acta Radiologica*. 2005 Jan 1;46(6):569–75.
7. Khafif A, Schneebaum S, Fliss DM, Lerman H, Metser U, Ben-Yosef R, Gil Z, Reider-Trejo L, Genadi L, Even-Sapir E. Lymphoscintigraphy for sentinel node mapping using a hybrid single photon emission CT (SPECT)/CT system in oral cavity squamous cell carcinoma. *Head & Neck*. 2006 Oct;28(10):874–9.

7

Histopathological Parameters for Prognosis of Disease

The prognosis of the disease mostly depends upon the various histopathological factors. These factors also help us plan the adjuvant treatment. The following are important factors for a clinician to have a clear microscopic idea of the disease.

Tumor Size

According to TNM staging classification, the size of a tumor is defined as the greatest surface dimension, also called tumor diameter. Many research articles in the literature have widely studied and described a correlation between metastasis and large tumor sizes at clinical presentation, which are most often associated with an increased risk of poor survival of a patient.

Risks of locally distant metastases for patients with tumors at stage T4 disease and those patients with more than one subsite involved are significantly higher in relation to those with tumors confined to the only one site or at early stage disease. It is also well understood that fewer bilateral metastases were found for T1 tumors compared with tumors that are more advanced primaries, and the patients with bilateral metastases had at least T2 disease or greater[1,2].

Tumor Thickness

Tumor thickness is usually examined by vertical measurement that is a line starting from the oral mucosa up to the deepest point of invasion with the help of a millimetric lens (0/20 mm). Both for invasive tumors and indurated or exophytic tumors, the upper point of the measurement is the line of oral mucosa. The thickness of a tumor is a direct micrometer measurement by the oncopathologist of the vertical bulk of the tumor irrespective of the histologic structure of the exophytic or an ulcerative form of tumor growth. At the same time, there are some studies on measuring the standard thickness of tumor or depth, which are controversial in English literature. This may be due to the fact that when the paraffin blocks are cut, they are not exactly of vertical depth. Tumor thickness is now widely recognized as a more accurate and apt histological prognosticator for cervical nodal metastasis, tumor local recurrence, and disease-free survival than tumor diameter[3]. Akheel et al.[3] performed a meta-analysis in 983 patients and concluded that tumor infiltration depth is an important prognosticator in pT1/pT2 cN0 necks. Tumors with depth of infiltration >4.5 mm, clinically or radiologically, should undergo elective neck dissection to improve the prognosis of head and neck squamous cell carcinoma (HNSCC).

Surgical Margin Status

The surgical margins of the tumor often include both the oral mucosal surface at the edge of the primary tumor and the submucosal layer and deeper connective tissues surrounding the primary tumor. The identification of tumor cells at resected surgical margins has been thought to be one of the most important prognosticators in OSCC patients. Many research studies have also suggested that total excision of a primary tumor with an adequate/sufficient surgical margin is an important point to consider. Even the relative risk of mortality associated with a close margin is similar to that associated with lymph nodal metastasis.

DOI: 10.1201/9780367822019-7

In recent English literature, Nason et al. found that the impact of disease-free survival improved with each additional millimeter of clear surgical margin, as every 1-mm increase in clear surgical margin decreased the risk of death of 5 years by 8%. On univariate correlation analysis for metastases of contralateral neck, many authors have studied and demonstrated that surgical margins had a significant statistical association with a high risk of developing contralateral lymph nodal metastases. Thereby, the accurate definition of the clear or close surgical margin is an important prognosticator when considered for planning adjunctive treatments for certain patients with oral SCC.

Histological margin is called an involved margin when there is invasive carcinoma and/or carcinoma in situ present on the surgical margins of the mucosa and/or the distance is 5 mm between the primary tumor and the normal mucosal margin. According to UK guidelines, the status of both the mucosal margin and deep margin and surgical margins of 5 mm are to be considered clear margins, 1–5 mm as close margin, and less than 1 mm as involved margin. Woolgar et al. stated in his study that even 5-mm margin may not be considered to be clear when the invasive pattern of tumor is not favorable with widely located satellites of tumors. However, in a study done retrospectively based on a historical cohort of 277 patients who were managed surgically with OSCC, Nason et al. suggested that an insufficient or close margin is a margin less than 3 mm of the marked resection margin. The widely accepted definition of a close margin of within 5 mm needs to be reconsidered. The shrinkage effect of surgical specimens must be considered ranging from 40% to 50%, when the tissues are fixed in formalin. It is widely thought that the margin after surgical resection with 1 cm or more of uninvolved tissue around the tumor is considered to be sufficient. Akheel et al., in 2019, conducted a meta-analysis in 1333 patients and concluded that margins of 5 mm are required to have a good prognosis of the patients and prevent local recurrences/death. A surgeon must concentrate on the surgical margins of at least 1–1.5 cm macroscopically to gain 5-mm clear microscopic pathological-free margins considering the shrinkage and tumor extent. A clear margin has recently been considered to provide sufficient management by surgery but this thinking has been challenged by numerous studies which pathologically document that clear or adequate margins do not always necessarily guarantee that the tumor cells are removed completely and patients with clear margins do not necessarily always have good clinical results, as 4%–18%[4] of tongue cancers with clear margins had local recurrence.

Hence, for an adequate resection surgical margin, there is no a single definition. Several variables, including the pattern of invasion of a tumor, thickness of a tumor, tumor satellites, tumor satellite distance, and other clinical factors, must be considered.

Parameters of Cervical (Regional) Lymph Nodes

Since many decades, the importance of prognostic factors such as the presence and extent of metastasis of cervical lymph nodes in SCC of oral cavity has been recognized. Numerous independent studies have reported a strong association between occurrences of lymph node metastasis, but there is no general agreement on what features the prognosis depends on. In relation to several features of cervical lymph node, the level and number of metastasis to ipsilateral lymph node has been investigated widely while extracapsular spread (ECS) has been commonly confirmed and reported by Kowalski et al. Patients who have ipsilateral metastatic cervical lymph nodes possess a very high risk of metastases to the contralateral lymph nodes of about 4.8 times higher when compared with the patients who have no metastases on the ipsilateral neck. Many other authors have further investigated that the patients having multiple ipsilateral positive lymph nodes of more than two present with a greater risk for contralateral or bilateral lymph node metastases as compared with those with a single positive or negative lymph node.

The extent of ECS is labeled "macroscopic" and "microscopic," when it is clearly found on pathological inspection and is most evident on assessment histologically. Several studies have emphasized on the prognostic importance of ECS and it is commonly identified/accepted as a sensitive, simple, and highly discriminating indicator.

Histological Grading

The OSCC histological grading is adopted by the Broder's/WHO grading system that recommends the following three categories:

- Grade 1 is well differentiated.
- Grade 2 is moderately differentiated.
- Grade 3 is poorly differentiated. It is based upon the consideration of a subjective assessment of the nuclear and cellular pleomorphism, degree of keratinization, and mitotic activity. Several authorities have now recognized that the poor correlation between prognosis and management response as shown in Broder's/WHO grade in an individual patient. It is mainly due to the lack of discrimination inherent in Broder's/WHO grading system: Around 90% of oral and oropharyngeal tumors are grade 2.

Tumor Invasion Pattern

To avoid some of the hindrances encountered in by the Broder's/WHO grading system, Jakobbson et al. put forward a grading system upon considering the multifactorial histological malignancy, which is considered simple but has multiple features of both the tumor cells and the interface between the host tissues and the tumor cells. Subsequently, there were many modifications made to search for a better histologic prognosticator to favor the outcome of OSCC patients. Bryne et al. and Anneroth et al. put forward a new grading system that was based on the pattern of tumor invasion (POI) from the margins deeper in tumor to connective tissues surrounding them. This system includes the following four categories:

1. Grade 1 tumors have borders that push outward with well-defined delineations.
2. Grade 2 tumors have advancing fronts with solid cords, bands, and strands.
3. Grade 3 tumors have groups or cords of infiltrating islands of tumor that consist of more than 15 cells on every island that are identified in the invasive border.
4. Grade 4 tumors have an obvious dissociation of tumor cells in small groups, which is less than 15 cells on every island and is situated at the main tumor interface and the surrounding tissues. Several independent authors have concluded that POI shows better prognostic values when compared with the conventional Broder's/WHO grading system in predicting patient's nodal metastasis, local recurrence, and survival.

Tumor Satellites and Tumor Satellite Distance

Tumor satellites are defined as separate islands of tumor cells of any size that have intervening normal healthy tissues at the tumor and nontumor interface. It has been reported that tumor satellite distance can also serve as a significant prognosticator of oral SCC. It has been reported in literature that microsatellite cells of tumor can spread up to 1–1.8 cm; these microscopic tumor cells that are often located at the deep mucosal margin are invisible and not readily palpable during surgery. Hence, these tumors may leave behind some distant tumor satellite cells beyond the surgical margins and lead to consequently local tumor recurrence, metastatic to cervical nodes, and then poor outcomes when surgical margins are imagined to be clear macroscopically. Yang et al. stated that tumor satellites that were seen in 92% of tumors were significantly related with a habit of tobacco chewing. Patients with tumor satellite distance greater or less than 0.5 mm had a statistical significance for better prognosis while the patients with tumor satellite distance greater than 0.5 mm had a greater incidence of local recurrence of tumor, shorter intervals to neck recurrence, and a very high propensity for metastasis to contralateral or bilateral cervical nodal metastasis.

Lymphovascular Invasion

Lymphovascular invasion (LVI), as proposed by Jakobbson et al., is a part of the multifactorial grading system and is classified based on the presence or absence of tumor cells that are located both in the wall and in the light of the lymphatic vessels or blood that imply an increasing likelihood of successful metastatic growth. It is difficult to recognize and define with certainty while considering the presence and extent of LVI. It has been studied that LVI has a significant co-relation with tumor size and thickness, tumor site, perineural invasion (PNI), histological grading and pattern of invasion, cervical nodal metastasis, local recurrence and status of surgical margins, and survival of the patient. Kowalski et al., in his study, suggested the presences of LVI and of PNI were significantly related to greater rates of risks of metastases in oral SCCs.[5]

Perineural Invasion

The definition of PNI is very similar to LVI, which is considered the presence of tumor tissue adjacent to the peri- or intratumoral nerves. Several previous researchers have put forward that this is a very valuable prognosticator for metastases in the neck. Its correlation with contralateral neck metastases in OSCC has been analyzed in a few research studies. González-García et al.[6] reported that PNI of the primary OSCC tumor was highly predictive for metastasis. It was confirmed by the presence of pathologic lymph neck nodes on the contralateral side in 17.02% of patients with PNI, while only 4.1% of those patients were without PNI.

Muscular Infiltration

Muscular infiltration is another important factor, which is measured in an objective manner. It tells us of the presence or absence of tumoral cells observed close to either the mucosal surface or deeper muscular tissue. It has been reported to be a very reliable and efficient predictive factor of metastasis of lymph node. A few studies described that it is not an important prognostic factor. Byers et al. studied and concluded that there is increased probability of occult metastasis if the invasion of the muscle exceeded for more than 4 mm. Pimmenta Amaral et al. found that the infiltration of muscle showed a very high probability of occult metastasis with lower disease-free survival in tumors that are located in the tongue and floor of the mouth in the initial stages.

Desmoplastic Reaction and Peritumoral Inflammation

A few studies have observed that peritumoral inflammation and desmoplastic reaction are significant factors for the prediction of cervical metastasis. González-García et al.[6] studied that peritumoral inflammation was much more significant in relation to metastasis in a study done in 203 patients in a retrospective analysis with SCC of the tongue. They have provided a clear explanation for this relation that it can happen when there is a low host immunological response around the primary tumor that could allow easier dissemination of tumor cells through lymphatic drainage[6].

A good histopathological report must cover all the histopathological parameters. A sample is provided below.

GROSS:

Received a specimen of right hemimandibulectomy measuring 11.0 × 5.0 × 4.5 cm with mandible measuring 10.0 cm in length.

An ulceroinfiltrative tumor is identified measuring 4.2 × 2.5 × 2.0 cm, involving right lower gingivo lingual sulcus.

On serial sectioning the maximum thickness of the tumor is 2.0 cm.

The underlying mandibular bone is grossly free of tumor.

The distance of various cut margins from the tumor are:

1.0 cm from anterior mucosal margin.
0.9 cm from posterior mucosal margin.

0.2 cm from medial mucosal margin.
0.9 cm from lateral mucosal margin.
0.2 cm from medial soft tissue cut margin.

1.1 cm from anterior bony cut margin.

Lymph Nodes:

[i] Right Level Ib lymph node (Along main specimen) -4 lymph nodes identified, largest measures 1.1 cm in diameter. Cut surface : Grayish white. Salivary gland measures 4.0 × 3.0 × 2.0 cm. Cut surface : Unremarkable.

[ii] Right Level II To IV lymph nodes - 7 lymph nodes identified, largest measures 1.2 cm in diameter. Cut surface : Unremarkable.

SECTIONS:

A,B & C - Tumor with medial soft tissue cut margin.
D - Anterior and posterior mucosal cut margin.
E - Tumor with medial mucosal cut margin.
F - Lateral mucosal cut margin.
G,H,I & J - Right Level Ib lymph node.
K,L,M & N - Right Level II to IV lymph nodes.
O - Underlying bone.
P - Anterior bony cut margin.

MICROSCOPIC (A to P):

Specimen type : Right hemimandibulectomy.

Moderately differentiated squamous cell carcinoma of right lower gingivo lingual sulcus.

Lymphovascular emboli are not seen.

Perineural invasion is not seen.

Medial mucosal cut margin is 0.2 cm away and is free of tumour.

Rest all the mucosal cut margins (Anterior, Posterior, Lateral) are free of tumour.

Medial soft tissue cut margin is 0.2 cm away and is free of tumour.

Lymph Nodes:

[i] Right Level Ib lymph node (along main specimen) - [2/4] Two out of four lymph nodes show metastatic deposits of squamous cell carcinoma without perinodal. Salivary gland is unremarkable.

[ii] Right Level II to IV lymph modes - [0/7] All seven lymph nodes are reactive and free of tumor.

IMPRESSION:

Specimen type : Right hemimandibulectomy.

MODERATELY DIFFERENTIATED SQUAMOUS CELL CARCINOMA OF RIGHT LOWER GINGIVO LINGUAL SULCUS WITH METASTATIC IPSILATERAL REGIONAL LYMPH NODES. STAGE - IVA [T3, N2].

AWAIT COMMENT ON UNDERLYING BONE AND BONY CUT MARGINS.

Prepared by
SADHAN KULSHRESHTHA

DR. Priyanka Sachdev M.D.   Dr. Qutbuddin Chahwala M.D.
Surgical Pathologist   Surgical Pathologist
REG:MP-11615   Reg:MP-3370

REFERENCES

1. Janot F, Klijanienko J, Russo A, Mamet JP, De Braud F, El-Naggar AK, Pignon JP, Luboinski B, Cvitkovic E. Prognostic value of clinicopathological parameters in head and neck squamous cell carcinoma: a prospective analysis. *British Journal of Cancer.* 1996 Feb;73(4):531–8.
2. Crissman JD, Liu WY, Gluckman JL, Cummings G. Prognostic value of histopathologic parameters in squamous cell carcinoma of the oropharynx. *Cancer.* 1984 Dec 15;54(12):2995–3001.
3. Akheel M, George RK, Jain A, Chahwala Q, Wadhwania A. Depth of tumor infiltration as a prognosticator in pT1-2 cN0 oral squamous cell carcinoma thereby need for elective neck dissection—a meta-analysis. *Cancer Research, Statistics, and Treatment.* 2019 Jan 1;2(1):61.
4. Akheel M, George RK, Jain A, Chahwala Q, Wadhwania A. Surgical margins and nodal metastasis are prognostic factors in oral squamous cell carcinoma: a meta-analysis. *Clinical Cancer Investigation Journal.* 2019 Mar 1;8(2):47.
5. Willen R, Nathanson A, Moberger G, Anneroth G. Squamous cell carcinoma of the gingiva: histological classification and grading of malignancy. *Acta Oto-Laryngologica.* 1975 Jan 1;79(1–2):146–54.
6. González-García R, Naval-Gías L, Román-Romero L, Sastre-Pérez J, Rodríguez-Campo FJ. Local recurrences and second primary tumors from squamous cell carcinoma of the oral cavity: a retrospective analytic study of 500 patients. *Head & Neck: Journal for the Sciences and Specialties of the Head and Neck.* 2009 Sep;31(9):1168–80.

8

Clinical Assessment of Head and Neck Cancer Patients

Clinical assessment of the patient with head and neck cancer (HNC) offers multiple and complex challenges for the surgeon. A comprehensive and systematic examination of the patient is required. A complete and thorough medical history of the patient should be taken, with special attention to key factors such as prior history of cancer; any habits like tobacco chewing, smoking, and intake of alcohol; extent of exposure of sun; gastric reflux; industrial or occupational exposures at work; and intake of immunosuppression drugs. Comorbidities of the patient must be documented due for many reasons: adverse impact on short-term mortality of patients with newly diagnosed HNSCC, reduced overall survival in HNSCC and possible predictor for distant metastases, adverse influence on disease-specific survival (DFS), probably due to the advanced stage at initial presentation of the disease and the likelihood of such patients undergoing less aggressive treatment, greater incidence of more severe complications, adverse impact on quality of life (QoL), adverse impact on functional and cosmetic outcomes, increased finance of treatment.

Important signs and symptoms are associated with HNSCC, pain, dysphagia, odynophagia, hoarseness or dysphonia, dyspnea, stridor, otalgia, other cranial nerve (CN) deficits, etc. Documentation of the clinical assessments must be performed that may influence the suitability of appropriate management such as resection of tumor surgically or radiation therapy. Critical and important information regarding any previous treatments must be collected, including previous oncologic surgeries, chemotherapy treatments, or prior radiotherapy.

A systematic examination of the HNC patient ideally involves major investigations like radiographic imaging such as CT/MRI scan and cytopathologic tissue analysis such as punch biopsy or fine needle aspiration (FNA) cytology.

A surgeon must perform comprehensive and thorough head and neck examination and any other additional physical examinations as indicated[1].

- Extract complete prior history and description of all symptoms.
- Ask for habits such as history of smoking, exposure to sun, radiation exposure, etc.
- Assess overall medical and functional status in the context of possible treatment options.
- Discuss with a paramedic head and neck team like cancer nurse, patient and family counselor, and a social worker to provide support and guidance to the patient.
- Note the critical information regarding prior therapies. Evaluate the airway for any urgent intervention: airway compromise, aspiration risk, obese neck, and trismus. If required an evaluation of risk factors from an anesthetist has to be taken for any prior difficult intubation, Mallampati grade III or IV, thyromental distance is less than 6 cm, limited mouth opening, inter-incisal distance is less than 3 cm, poor dentition, reduced extension of the neck, presence of retrognathia, tongue base tumor, obstructive laryngeal tumors, hypopharyngeal lesions, any previous head and neck surgery or radiotherapy.
- Obtain histopathological specimens for documentation and diagnosis.
- Recognize the patient's and their family's concerns about the diagnosis and acknowledge the impact regarding anxiety, stress, fear, and grief.
- Organize a multidisciplinary tumor board meeting and specialty referrals as indicated: medical oncology, radiation oncology, maxillofacial surgery/prosthodontics, speech and swallow therapy, anesthesiology/medicine, pain management, social work, financial/benefits counseling, smoking cessation resources.

DOI: 10.1201/9780367822019-8

- Order hematological examinations and other laboratory studies if required.
- Clearly identify and explain the next steps in diagnosis and manage in terms of appropriate for the individual patient and get a written consent signed by patient and relative that you have explained about the procedure and risks (important for medicolegal purpose).

Physical Examination

It is essential that a surgeon perform a thorough physical and head and neck evaluation of the patient that is essential, regardless of suspected primary site (Figure 8.1). In addition to clinical visualization and of normal anatomic structures of the head and neck region, manual palpation with a finger is a must and a critical tool for assessment of head and neck tumors (Figure 8.2). Finger palpation should be performed routinely while examining the oral cavity and neck. Bimanual palpation is necessary for detailed and comprehensive evaluation of the lesions/tumors on the floor of mouth and submandibular/sublingual areas. Palpation techniques can yield certain critical information regarding submucosal or bony fixation, extension, and thickness/induration of the tumor[2].

Examination and assessment of facial structures should be done to determine any facial swelling or gross asymmetry. A thorough external inspection of the patient's skin for any suspicious lesions should also be performed. External examination of the ear and temporal bone is a required portion of the clinical assessment. Inspection of the skin overlying the external ear and mastoid region and also palpated when there is an appropriate need. Following inspection of the external ear, otoscopic examination should be performed to assess the tympanic membrane, external auditory canal, and middle ear space.

Examination of nose must be done with anterior rhinoscopy under direct visualization with a headlight and a nasal speculum. With exposure enhanced by appropriate speculum technique, the anterior nasal cavity and its contents are visualized, including the vestibule, anterior septum, and floor of the nasal cavity, inferior turbinate, middle turbinate and middle meatus. Suspicion for any sinonasal mass/pathology, obstruction, secretions, scabbing, or active bleeding should be checked.

A thorough and systematic assessment of the oral cavity starts anteriorly with the lips from the skin/mucosal junction of the vermillion border. The junction of hard and soft palate, the anterior tonsillar pillar, and circumvallate papillae form a posterior plane separate the oral cavity from the oropharynx.

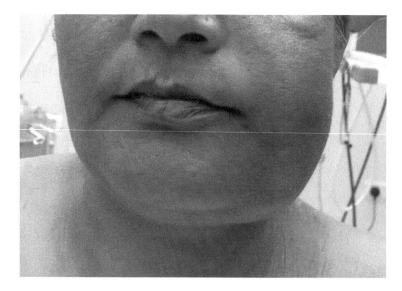

FIGURE 8.1   On inspection of this patient, there is facial asymmetry on the side of the left cheek with skin induration on palpation.

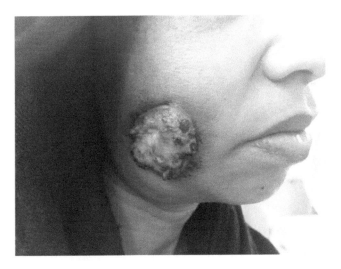

FIGURE 8.2 On inspection, there is a fungating mass of the right side of the cheek with inflamed borders.

The oral cavity is divided into the following anatomic subsites: the lips, floor of mouth, retromolar trigone (RMT), buccal mucosa, oral tongue, hard palate, and upper and lower alveolus (Figure 8.3).

Oral cavity examination is best performed with a tongue spatula and a headlight. When the patients open the mouth, the presence/absence of trismus must be noted as it might involve pterygoid muscles. The buccal mucosa, gingivobuccal sulci, gingiva, the RMT, and overall state of dentition are then examined. The oral tongue is then grasped with a piece of gauze and gently manipulated to check the ventral, dorsal, and lateral surfaces for any abnormality. All the surfaces must be inspected for any ulcers or lesions. The floor of mouth should be inspected and palpated manually and any lesions in FOM should raise a suspicion for minor salivary gland tumors. All movements of the tongue are tested to check any asymmetric protrusion for involvement of the cranial XII nerve.

Inspection and palpation of the hard palate are performed. Complete examination of the oral cavity requires assessment of all the mucosal surface changes that show any signs of potential or *premalignancy conditions* such as erythroplakia, leukoplakia, oral submucosal fibrosis, lichen planus, discoid lupus erythematosus, and dyskeratosis. The most common sites for these premalignant lesions include

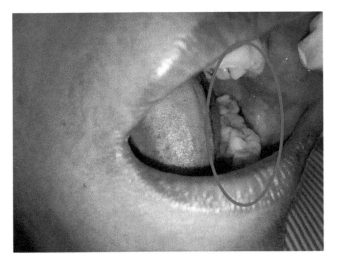

FIGURE 8.3 Intraoral examination shows a 3 × 2 cm ulcerative lesion in the left gingiva-buccal sulcus. Palpation is done with finger to check the induration of the lesion.

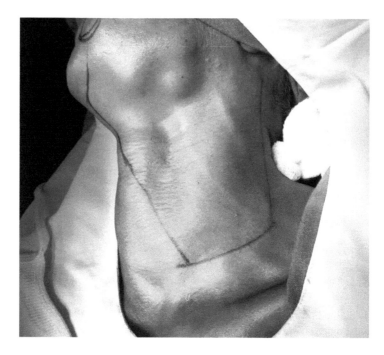

FIGURE 8.4 Palpation of the neck is important to check for any cervical lymphadenopathy. In this patient, a level IB lymph node is enlarged.

the buccal mucosa, tongue, lower gingiva, and floor of mouth. Additional screening methods, including application of toluidine blue, fluorescence, and brush biopsy technique, have not proven it must be of unequivocal benefit in enhancing detection of oral malignancy, but early findings regarding the potential application of optical coherence tomography in early detection yield promising results.

Examination of the neck in an HNSCC is paramount and most significant in the evaluation of HNC patients. All neck levels, including the supraclavicular region, should be palpated to assess for the presence of cervical lymphadenopathy (Figure 8.4). Size, mobility, and location of any suspected malignant lymph nodes should be carefully documented in relation to these levels. The thyroid gland should be examined and palpated for the presence of any solitary nodules or any gross enlargement. The parotid glands, the preauricular lymph nodes, and the postauricular lymph nodes should be palpated. A tumor in the parotid gland may represent primary neoplasm, metastatic lymph node, a cyst, or any inflammatory process. In cases where the primary lesion is not discovered (occult primary) on initial physical examination, further diagnostic workup with adjunctive imaging (CT, MRI, or PET/PET-CT), tissue sampling, operative endoscopy, and immunohistochemical or molecular studies as indicated will facilitate ultimate discovery of the primary lesion in 97% of patients. Classification of lymph node levels has been provided in the previous chapters.

A complete cranial assessment should be performed with a keen focus on the CNs. CN deficits may be indicators of underlying neoplastic processes and may require further additional workup. Any paresis of the facial nerve (CN VII) must be characterized in accordance with the House-Brackmann grading scale.

Fiberoptic endoscopy provides the most accurate and clear visualization of oropharynx, nasopharynx, and laryngeal areas, allowing for assessment of primary lesions and evaluation of airway status. Findings from physical examination considered in the context of a patient's symptomatology and risk factor profile form the basis for further workup. In most of the cases, a comprehensive evaluation of suspicious findings will require adjunctive imaging. Prior to any treatment, definitive tissue diagnosis must be obtained by FNA, core needle biopsy, or open biopsy. Operative endoscopy with biopsy may also assist in securing definitive tissue diagnosis and achieving accurate staging (Figure 8.5).

Head and neck cancer involves a heterogenous and varied group of pathologic neoplasms/tumors with a wide variation in accordance of histopathogenesis, tumor biology, required pretreatment workup, optimal

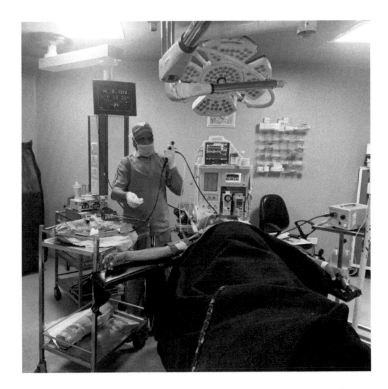

FIGURE 8.5 Operating room photo with an anesthetist holding the fiber optic laryngoscopy for a severe trismus patient diagnosed with carcinoma buccal mucosa with OSMF for intubation.

treatment modality, prognosis of the patient, and quality-of-life implications. Given this complexity, successful management of this disease process requires a concerted systematic multidisciplinary approach. Comprehensive treatment of HNC patients involves a keen participation by various specialists: head and neck surgeons, medical oncologists, radiation oncologists, head and neck pathologists, neuroradiologists, oral pathologists, facial plastic and microvascular reconstructive surgeons, endocrinologists, oral surgeons, dental pathologists, maxillofacial prosthodontists, speech pathologists, social workers, nutritionists, occupational therapists, nursing coordinators, research coordinators, nurses, and others. Coordinating such interdisciplinary care can be challenging but is necessary to furnish optimal patient care.

In most institutions, weekly/monthly head and neck tumor boards have emerged as the institutional protocol for coordinating the interdisciplinary care of head and neck cancer patients, and recent studies have the impact of multidisciplinary tumor boards on the provision of head and neck cancer care. In addition to providing a structured, regular mechanism for interdisciplinary collaboration, tumor boards also provide a forum for reevaluation of outside pathology and radiology findings. Evidence from English literature demonstrates multiple benefits from the routine engagement of multidisciplinary tumor board meetings, including improved staging accuracy, greater accordance with guidelines and clinical practice, improved communication between providers, enhanced cost-effectiveness of care, shorter time lapse from diagnosis to initiation of treatment, and improved clinician and patient satisfaction (Figure 8.6).

The complexity of the pathologic entities involved and the enormity of the potential impact on patients and their family members precludes the adoption of a facile approach to assessment and evaluation, treatment, or patient interaction. Head and neck abnormalities have profound effects on patients because, in addition to the cancer type, fundamental qualities of life are often affected, including facial appearance, facial identity, and important functions of living that includes breathing, speaking, and eating. Undertaking the treatment of patients with head and neck cancer demands that surgeons maintain both vigilance and vigor in providing the best possible care.

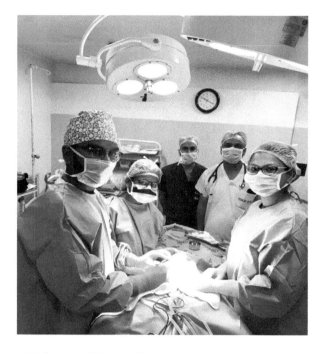

FIGURE 8.6 Maintaining OR decorum. HBSAg positive patient diagnosed with carcinoma buccal mucosa.

REFERENCES

1. Hornig JD, Malin BT, Oconnell B. Clinical evaluation of the head and neck cancer patient. *Head and neck cancer: a multidisciplinary approach*, Fourth Electronic Edition. Philadelphia, PA: LWW. 2014.
2. Robson A, Sturman J, Williamson P, Conboy P, Penney S, Wood H. Pre-treatment clinical assessment in head and neck cancer: United Kingdom National Multidisciplinary Guidelines. *Journal of Laryngology & Otology*. 2016 May;130(S2):S13–22.

9

Management of the Neck

Classification of neck dissection was standardized in 1991. Later, it was publicized by the Academy's Committee for Head and Neck Surgery and Oncology.

Academy Classification (1991)

1. Radical neck dissection (RND)
2. Modified RND (MRND)
3. Selective neck dissection (SND)
   - Supraomohyoid type
   - Lateral type
   - Posterolateral type
   - Anterior compartment type
4. Extended RND
5. RND is the standard procedure for cervical lymphadenectomy, that is, the removal of all cervical lymph nodes. All the other modifications are compared with RND
6. Modifications of the standard RND procedure include the preservation of all non-lymphatic structures are called MRND
7. Any type of neck dissection that preserves one or more groups or levels of lymph nodes is called an SND
8. An extended neck dissection is the excision of additional lymph nodal groups or non-lymphatic structures relative to the RND

Medina Classification (1989)

- Comprehensive neck dissection
- RND
- MRND
  - *Type I*: Preservation of spinal accessory nerve (SAN)
  - *Type II*: Preservation of SAN and internal jugular vein (IJV)
  - *Type III*: Preservation of SAN, IJV, and sternocleidomastoid (SCM)
- SND

Spiro Classification (1994)

- Radical (resection of four or five node levels)
- RND
- MRND

DOI: 10.1201/9780367822019-9

- Extended RND
- Modified and extended RND—selective (resection of three node levels)
- Supraomohyoid neck dissection (SOHND)
- Jugular dissection (lymph node levels II–IV)
- Any other three node levels resected
- Limited (resection of no more than two node levels)
- Paratracheal node dissection
- Mediastinal node dissection
- Any other one or two node levels resected

For incisions of neck dissection (refer to *Surgeon's Knife: Head and Neck Incisions* by Akheel Mohammad, Jaypee Medical Publishers, 2016).

Neck Dissections

"Neck dissection" refers to a surgical procedure that is carried out by resecting the lymphatic structures and also the fibro fatty tissue of the neck as part of the surgical protocol for the treatment of cervical lymphatic metastasis. As most malignancies of the upper aerodigestive tract mainly metastasize to the group of cervical lymph nodes, neck dissections must be performed with or without continuity with a surgical excision of these malignancies[1].

Radical Neck Dissection

Indications: When there is extensive cervical involvement or matted lymph nodes with gross extracapsular spread and invasion into the SAN, IJV, or SCM (Figure 9.1).

1. This surgical procedure is always done under general anesthesia; the patient is placed in a reverse Trendelenburg position with the extension of their neck at atlantoaxial joint and then the head is elevated 10 degrees above the table. The face must be positioned to the contralateral side of the surgical dissection with an extension of the neck.

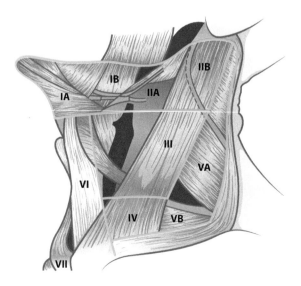

FIGURE 9.1   Radical neck dissection.

2. Operating site of the neck must be cleaned with Betadine scrub and then with Betadine solution two to three times; sterile draping of the operating site with towels over a polydrape sheet must be done to minimize infection rate.

3. Incision of choice for RND is Lahey's lateral utility incision in postirradiated patients. Modified Schobinger's incision is very useful in patients undergoing commando surgery. MacFee double horizontal incision can be used in these patients who have completed radiation.

4. Neck incision is marked with a surgical marker pen or with methylene blue and then infiltrated with 10- to 15-ml solution of 1% xylocaine with adrenaline of 1:80,000. Wait for at least five minutes and then make a skin incision with surgical blade no. 15, raise a flap subplatysmally superiorly until the lower border of the mandible is exposed, tip of mastoid posteriorly, midline of the neck anteriorly, anterior border of trapezius posteriorly, and inferiorly until the clavicle.

5. Then the clavicular part of SCM muscle is dissected with electrocautery about 2 cm above the clavicular bone after separating it from IJV very carefully. Dissect and separate the IJV from its fascial attachments with the vagus nerve and common carotid artery. The lower end of the IJV is ligated at the level of the common tendinous attachment of two bellies of the omohyoid muscle that cross the IJV above. Transfix the IJV after ligating with double ligatures. This is called the "Houseman suture". Retract the IJV gradually upward along with the SCM muscle after holding them with Babcock forceps.

6. Dissect all the lymph nodes very carefully without damaging them, lymphatics and fat and fascia from the supraclavicular fossa along with level V lymph nodes. Utmost care must be taken to not cause any damage to the phrenic nerve, the brachial plexus, and transverse cervical vessels. The greater auricular nerve (GAN) passes at the junction of the upper 1/3 and lower 2/3 of SCM muscle, which is seen exiting from cervical plexus crossing the posterior border of external jugular vein (EJV). The GAN winds around the posterior border of the SCM muscle traveling upward and obliquely to enter into the tail of the parotid salivary gland. The SAN also exits at this particular point now, which is referred to as Erb's point, and runs within the posterior triangle of the neck to enter into the trapezius muscle.

7. Both nerves have to be dissected carefully from their cutaneous branches supplying the fascia and skin. At a level of thyroid cartilage, ligate the middle thyroid vein and resect all the lymph nodes along the middle 1/3 of the IJV, thereby clearing levels III and IV.

8. Now at the upper end of IJV, dissection at the extent of level of posterior belly of digastric can be the ideal landmark for ligating the upper end of the IJV. The transverse process of atlas can be considered a bony landmark. Place the double ligatures and then transfix it with a 3-0 silk suture and dissect the IJV after ligating the venae commitante for the hypoglossal nerves. This will clear level IIA and IIB lymph nodes.

9. The next step is the dissection of level IA and IB nodes along with submandibular salivary glands. A complete removal of the specimen en bloc is expected to be done. Irrigate the dissected field with normal saline and dilute Betadine and saline solution. After securing a complete hemostasis, place a Romo Vac drain of 14–16 FG size drain, fix it with braided silk sutures or a free tie, and then connect it to the drain box. After repositioning the skin flap, the first layer of muscle is sutured with 3-0 vicryl or catgut suture and then the skin is closed with staples or 3-0 Ethicon sutures. Apply pressure dressing and check whether the drain function is charged completely before extubating the patient or when required the ET tube can be kept electively for one day and the patient can be extubated the next day.

10. Postoperatively, the patient is kept in Fowler's position and given IV antibiotics for 3–5 days. The suction drain is removed when collection is less than 10 ml. The patient can be discharged on 5th–7th day and the sutures can be removed on 12th–14th postoperative day. Patient follow-up is done after 10 days, check the histopathology report for the need of any adjuvant therapy, which can be started after one month from the date of surgery. Contrast CT scan or PET-CT scan should be advised after a 6-month follow-up to check for the status of disease.

11. One monthly follow-up continues for 1 year; thereafter, 3 months for 2 years and then 6 months for 5 years.

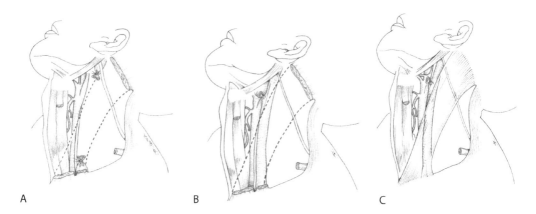

A   B   C

FIGURE 9.2   MRND: (A) type I, (B) type II, and (C) type III.

Modified Neck Dissection (Figure 9.2)

Definition
- Resection of lymph node-bearing areas as in RND with the preservation of one or more non-lymphatic structures that is IJV, SAN, or SCM.
- Non-lymphatic structures that are spared are specifically named in brackets.
- MRND is analogous to the "functional neck dissection" described by Bocca et al.

Medina et al. in 1989 described three types of modifications, commonly referred to, not specifically named by committee.

- *Type I*: SAN is preserved
- *Type II*: SAN and IJV are preserved
- *Type III*: SAN, IJV, and SCM ("functional neck dissection") are preserved

Procedure
1. The basic procedure of neck dissection shall remain the same as RND, but surgeon must preserve one/more than one of the three non-lymphatic structures, i.e., SAN, SCM muscle, and IJV. Preserve the transverse cervical vessels and GAN for decreased morbidity.

Rationale
- It has reduced postsurgical shoulder dysfunction (frozen shoulder syndrome) and shoulder pain.
- Improves cosmetic outcome and results.
- It reduces the likelihood of bilateral IJV resection in a patient with bilateral lymph node metastasis.

Selective Neck Dissection

Definition
- Defined as a cervical lymphadenectomy with the preservation of one or more groups of lymph nodes.

- There are common subtypes:
  - SOHND
  - Posterolateral neck dissection (PLND)
  - Lateral neck dissection (LND)
  - Anterior neck dissection (AND)

It is also known as an elective neck dissection (END). The rate of occult metastasis is 20–30% in clinically (N0) negative neck.

Indication: Primary lesion having 20% or greater risk for occult metastasis.

Studies done by Fisch and Sigel (1964) demonstrated systematic and predictable routes of lymphatic spread from mucosal surfaces of the head and neck. Depending upon the surgeon's decision to upgrade the neck intraoperatively, frozen sections needed to confirm squamous cell carcinoma (SCC) in suspicious lymph nodes (Rassekh et al.) for the need for post-op radiation therapy.

Procedure
1. Modified Schobinger incision or Apron flap incision is among the best incisions for this surgical procedure. Dissection of lymph node will start from level I and will go to level III/IV in SOHND and will include level VI in anterior compartment lymph node dissection.

Supraomohyoid Neck Dissection (SOHND) (Figure 9.3)

This is the most commonly performed SND.

Definition
- It is defined as en bloc removal of level I–III cervical lymph node groups.
- Posterior border of the SCM and cervical plexus forms the posterior unit.
- Inferior limit is the omohyoid muscle overlying the IJV.

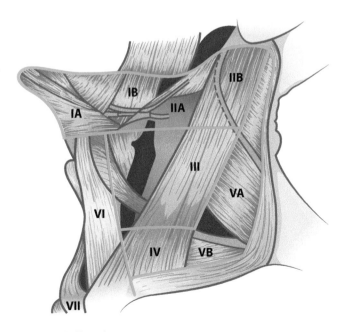

FIGURE 9.3 Supraomohyoid neck dissection.

Rationale

- Expectant management of the N0 neck is not advised
- Based on Lindberg's study in 1972
  - Distribution of lymph node metastasis in head and neck SCC
  - Subdigastric and midjugular lymph nodes are mostly affected in oral cavity carcinomas
  - Level IV and V lymph nodes are rarely involved

Lateral Type SND (Figure 9.4)

Definition
- Defined as en bloc removal of the level II–IV jugular lymph nodes.

Indications: For N0 neck in carcinomas of the oropharynx, hypopharynx, supraglottis, and larynx.

Posterolateral Type SND

Definition

- Defined as en bloc resection of lymph node-bearing tissues in levels II–IV and some additional node groups like a suboccipital and postauricular.

Indications

- Malignancies of cutaneous origin like SCC, Merkel cell carcinoma, and melanoma.
- Soft tissue sarcomas of the neck and scalp.

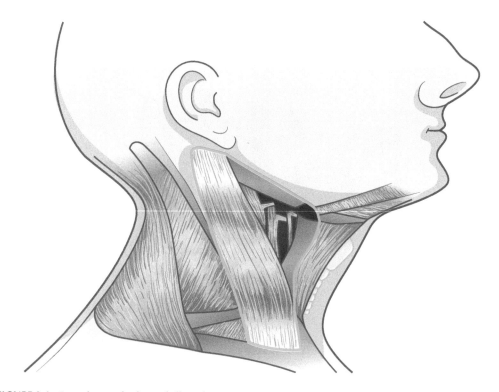

FIGURE 9.4   Lateral type selective neck dissection.

Anterior Compartment SND

Definition

- Defined as en bloc resection of level VI lymph structures in level VI
- Perithyroidal nodes
- Pretracheal nodes
- Precricoid nodes or Delphian
- Paratracheal nodes along recurrent nerves
- Limits of the dissection are the hyoid bone, suprasternal notch, and carotid sheaths

Indications

- Parathyroid carcinoma
- Subglottic carcinoma
- Laryngeal carcinoma with subglottic extension
- Carcinoma of the cervical esophagus
- Selected cases of thyroid carcinoma

Extended Neck Dissection (END)

Definition

- Any previous neck dissection that includes the removal of one or more additional lymph node groups and/or non-lymphatic structures.
- Usually performed with N+ necks in MRND or RND when there are metastases in structures that are usually preserved.

Indications

- Invasion of carotid artery
- Other examples are:
  - Resection of the hypoglossal nerve resection or digastric muscle
  - Dissection of central compartment and mediastinal nodes for subglottic involvement
  - Retropharyngeal lymph nodes are removed for tumors originating in the pharyngeal walls

Complications of Neck Dissection

Complications of neck dissection are often broadly divided into early, intermediate, and late.

Immediate Complications[2]

Hemorrhage: After the surgery, the most common complication is postoperative hemorrhage. External bleeding from the surgical incision site often originates from a blood vessel located subcutaneously. Often in these types of patients, it may be easily controlled by direct cauterization with electrocautery or infiltration of anesthetic solution in the surrounding tissues containing epinephrine or by ligation with free tie or nylon sutures. Persistent swelling or ballooning of the skin flaps that cause rising from the surgical bed immediately after surgical procedure with or without evidence of external bleeding must be attributed to a wound hematoma. If this hematoma is detected early and if the suctions drains are working well without blockage, then immediate evacuation of the accumulated blood must be done to resolve the problem. If this is not addressed immediately or if blood re-accumulates quickly beneath the skin flaps, it is thereby appropriate to return the patient back to the operating room and reexplore the surgical wound under strict aseptic conditions, thereby evacuating the hematoma and identifying the bleeding vessel and control the bleeding.

Airway obstruction: In cases of bilateral neck dissections for a tumor crossing midline, it may be associated with soft tissue edema. Moreover, any kind of resection of the primary malignant upper aerodigestive may also increase the edema of the upper airway. It is always good to be prepared with all necessary surgical instruments to carry out elective tracheotomy whenever required to protect the airway. A surgeon must be experienced to carry out tracheostomy.

Increased intracranial pressure: The intracranial pressure usually rises when the IJV is ligated during neck dissection. When IJV ligation is done, the pressure rises by threefold, and when both IJV are ligated, it increases by fivefold. This is usually temporary and the pressure will normalize within 24 hours. If it persists for more than 24–48 hours, head end elevation, steroids, and mannitol are often used.

Nerve injury: The important nerves that are at risk of injury during neck dissection are the phrenic nerve, vagus nerve, SAN, lingual nerve, and hypoglossal nerve. SAN injury causes difficulty in shrugging shoulders called frozen shoulder syndrome and shoulder hand syndrome. Injury to hypoglossal nerve will cause paralysis of tongue. Injury to the vagus nerve may manifest as voice problems and aspiration. Injury to the phrenic nerve leads to paradoxical breathing and lingual nerve injury can cause taste problems. Nerve injury called neuropraxia may recover within months whereas neurotmesis and axonotmesis have varying clinical outcomes.

Carotid sinus syndrome: This happens due to undue manipulation and excess pressure on the carotid sinus baroreceptors. It may result in hypotension and bradycardia. Scarring postoperatively may also make the sinus receptor sensitive turning the head and even cause palpation.

Pneumothorax: Neck dissection is much lower in the neck while resecting the level IV lymph nodes might cause injury to the apical part of lung pleura, which may lead to pneumothorax. The patient may become cyanosed, restless, and dyspnoeic after surgery. A plain radiograph of the chest most often provides the diagnosis. Emphysema, which may be minimal, may resolve itself whereas severe cases may require intercostal chest drains (ICDs).

Intermediate Complications

Pulmonary complications: Basal collapse and bronchopneumonia may occur in those patients who are smokers and in patients having preexisting chronic obstructive lung disease.

Deep vein thrombosis: This is seen in patients of elderly age and had surgeries that last for a long duration, patients who are prolonged bedridden, and patients with a past history of pulmonary embolism, deep vein thrombosis, thrombophilia, and myocardial infarction.

Chylous fistula: This often occurs due to the injury of the thoracic duct while performing a RND in the lower neck or mediastinum behind the IJV on the left side. If chylous fistula is suspected, every attempt must be made to suture it during the surgery by identifying it by head-down position and performing a modified Valsalva maneuver. It should be anticipated when the drain collection is milky in nature and increases dramatically by volume. Daily pressure dressings and a fat-restricted diet are the form of conservative management for chyle leak. When the collection of drain reaches 600 ml per day or more, it is an immediate indication for the reexploration of the wound and repair of the injured thoracic duct under with/without a microscope.

Carotid artery rupture: This usually occurs when the skin wound breaks down because of previous irradiation, secondary infection, and poor metabolic condition of the patient. It is mostly a fatal and deadly complication leading to imminent mortality if not intervened immediately. Control of bleeding by immediate finger pressure, airway management, blood transfusion, and exploration in operation theater has to be done.

Late Complications

- *Recurrence*: Recurrence can be at the primary tumor site, in the lymph nodes, or as a distant metastasis in the lung, liver, and brain
- *Lymph edema*: When the ligation of both the IJVs is done, lymphedema often follows owing to interruption of the lymphatic drainage channels from the head
- *Hypertrophic scars*
- *Parotid tail hypertrophy*
- *Hypothyroidism*

REFERENCES

1. Shah JP, Montero PH. New AJCC/UICC staging system for head and neck, and thyroid cancer. *Revista Médica Clínica Las Condes*. 2018 Jul 1;29(4):397–404.
2. Watkinson J, Gilbert R. *Stell & Maran's textbook of head and neck surgery and oncology*. CRC Press; 2011 Dec 30.

10

Access Osteotomies

DOI: 10.1201/9780367822019-10

History

In 1859, Von Langenbeck first performed a LeFort I maxillary osteotomy for the removal of a benign nasopharyngeal polyp. Curioni, Clauser, and Janecka introduced the concept of craniofacial dismantling and reassembly in the management of skull base tumors. Since then, many surgical approaches have been developed and refined using both pedicled as well as nonpedicled access osteotomies.

Mandibular Access Osteotomies

Mandibular access osteotomies are indicated for:

- Retromaxillary/Posterior maxillary lesions
- Posterior oral cavity lesions
- Parapharyngeal lesions
- Lateral pharyngeal lesions
- Deep space lesions of the neck

Access osteotomies may include median or paramedian osteotomy (Figure 10.1). It can be a step or vertical mandibulotomy with a mandibular swing approach. This osteotomy can be done at the symphysis and parasymphysis regions anterior to the mental foramen to preserve the neurovascular structures. During mandibulotomy with symphysis, stripping of genioglossus, anterior belly of digastrics, geniohyoid is done. The advantage of parasymphysis osteotomy is that it avoids the need for dissecting all these muscles. This osteotomy, if done in the form of a step, improves the stability of the mandible after osteosynthesis[1,3].

Ramus Osteotomy

This is performed to access parapharyngeal, tongue-based, and posterior maxilla tumors (Figure 10.2).

1. Inverted "L" osteotomy
2. Lateral segment osteotomy
3. Vertical subsigmoid osteotomy

Mandibular Swing Approach (Attia Approach)

For increased exposure of the parapharyngeal space, infratemporal fossa and pterygomaxillary region up to the skull base with this approach, a second horizontal osteotomy above the lingual of the mandibular ramus may be necessary. This anterolateral approach was originally described by Attia in 1984. Its

Parasymphyseal
osteotomy

Symphyseal
mandibulotomy

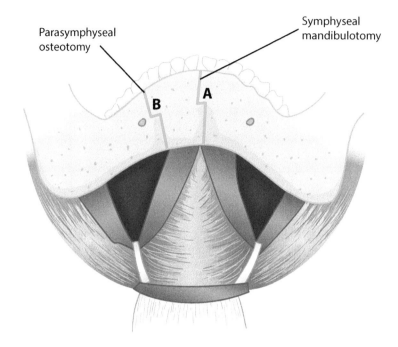

FIGURE 10.1   Symphyseal and parasymphyseal mandibulotomy.

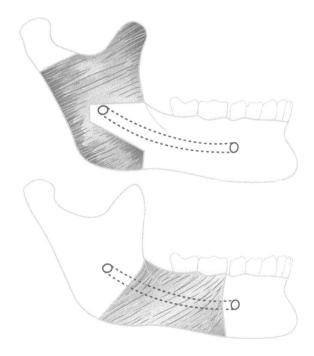

FIGURE 10.2   Ramus osteotomy and lateral segment osteotomy.

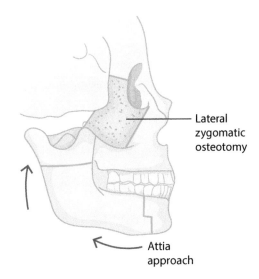

FIGURE 10.3 Lateral zygomatic (midface) osteotomy and Attia approach.

disadvantage is the need for tracheostomy. Smith et al. proposed that the access to the parapharyngeal space can be improved by vertical ramus osteotomy with a parasymphyseal mandibulotomy[2,3] (Figures 10.3 and 10.4).

Midface and Lateral Zygomatic Osteotomies

Zygomatic osteotomies are indicated for the following:

1. Posterior maxillary lesions
2. Retromaxillary lesions
3. Nasopharyngeal lesions

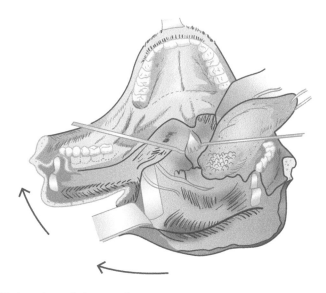

FIGURE 10.4 Mandibular swing or Attia approach.

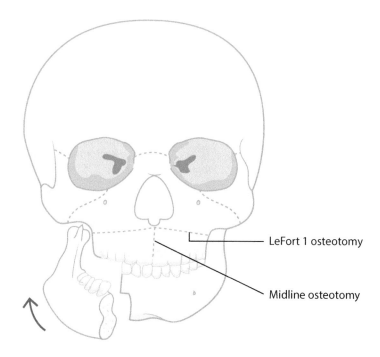

FIGURE 10.5   LeFort I midface osteotomy.

(For head and neck incisions, refer to *Surgeon's Knife: Head and Neck Incisions* by Akheel Mohammad, Jaypee Medical Publishers, 2016.)

Maxillofacial access osteotomies facilitate easy and complete removal of lesions in the head and neck region without damaging the adjacent vital structures (Figure 10.5). This approach is safe and simple and is associated with shorter operation time. The advent of low-profile mini-plates and screws has made the reestablishment of facial skeletal anatomy easier and faster. These access osteotomies form a major factor for decreasing morbidity rates. A multidisciplinary team approach including maxillofacial surgeons is often required with a systematic planning for the removal of hidden lesions of the head and neck[2,3].

REFERENCES

1. Devireddy SK, Kishore KR, Gali RS, Kanubaddy SR, Dasari MR, Akheel M. Access osteotomies of maxillofacial region: a report of three cases. *Archives of International Surgery.* 2013 May 1;3(2):193.
2. Devireddy SK, Kumar RK, Gali R, Kanubaddy SR, Dasari MR, Akheel M. Mucormycotic skull base osteomyelitis: a case report. *Journal of Oral and Maxillofacial Surgery, Medicine, and Pathology.* 2014;26(3):336–9.
3. McGregor IA, McGregor FM. *Cancer of the face and mouth: pathology and management for surgeons.* Churchill Livingstone; 1986.

11

Oral Cavity and Lips

TNM Classification

Primary tumor (T)

- *TX*: Primary tumor cannot be assessed
- *T0*: No evidence of primary tumor
- *Tis*: Carcinoma in situ
- *T1*: 2 cm or less in dimension
- *T2*: >2 cm to <4 cm in dimension and depth of induration (DOI) ≤ 10 mm or tumor ≤2 cm and DOI > 5 mm ≤ 10 mm
- *T3*: >4 cm in dimension, tumor of any size and DOI > 10 mm
- *T4*: Invade to cortical bone, inferior alveolar nerve (IAN), floor of mouth (FOM), skin of face
- *T4a*: Invading adjacent structure
- *T4b*: Invade pterygoid plates (PP), masticator space (MS), skull base, and internal carotid artery (ICA)

Regional lymph node (N) (Figure 11.1)

- *NX*: Lymph nodes cannot be assessed
- *N0*: No lymph node metastasis is seen
- *N1*: Single ipsilateral node <3 cm in dimension
- *N2*: Single ipsilateral node >3 cm to <6 cm
- *N2a*: Single ipsilateral node >3 cm to <6 cm
- *N2b*: Multiple ipsilateral node <6 cm
- *N2c*: B/L or contralateral node <6 cm in dimension
- *N3*: Node >6 cm

Distant metastasis (M)

- *MX*: Metastasis cannot be assessed
- *M0*: No distant metastasis
- *M1*: Distant metastasis

TNM Staging

- *Stage 0*: Tis N0 M0
- *Stage I*: T1 N0 M0
- *Stage II*: T2 N0 M0
- *Stage III*: T3 N0 M0
  - T1 N1 M0
  - T2 N1 M0
  - T3 N1 M0

DOI: 10.1201/9780367822019-11

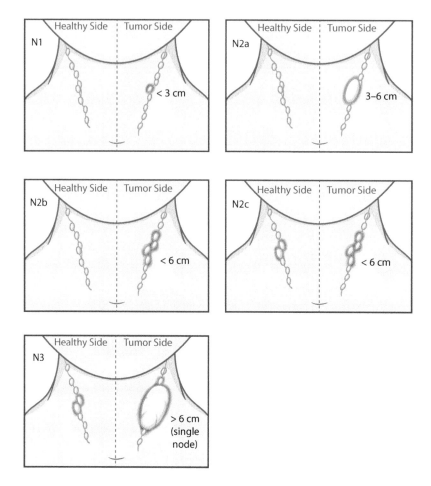

FIGURE 11.1   Nodal classification.

- *Stage IVA*: T4a N0 M0
  - T4a N1 M0
  - T1 N2 M0
  - T2 N2 M0
  - T3 N2 M0
  - T4a N2 M0
- *Stage IVB*: Any T N3 M0
  - T4b any N M0
- *Stage IVC*: Any T Any N M1

Pathways of Spread

Carcinoma Buccal Mucosa

Most primary buccal squamous cell carcinomas are confined to the mucosal layer during the early stages of spread (Figure 11.2). As the disease progresses, carcinoma infiltrates the underlying submucosa, muscle and extends submucosally and posteriorly along the buccinator muscle to the pterygomandibular

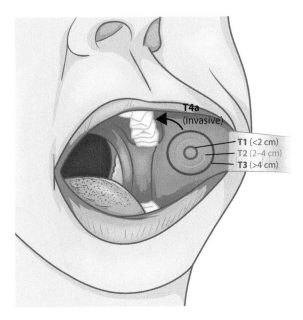

FIGURE 11.2 Carcinoma buccal mucosa.

raphe, which is considered the most common anatomical area for spread and anteriorly to the orbicularis oris and lip. Following this infiltrative growth, buccal squamous cell carcinomas might extend to the subcutaneous fat tissue and dermis to involve the skin of the cheek[1].

Management

1. *Wide excision (intraoral)*: For T1 and T2 lesion and not involving upper and lower gingivobuccal sulcus
2. *Wide excision (extraoral)*: For T2–T4 lesion involving upper and lower gingivobuccal sulcus or mandible

Reconstructive options include

1. *Local flaps*: Buccal fat pad, nasolabial flaps, tongue flap
2. *Regional flaps*: Pectoralis major myocutaneous flap/submental flaps/deltopectoral flap
3. *Distant flaps*: Free radial artery forearm flap/anterolateral thigh flap

Carcinoma of the Tongue

Squamous cell carcinomas occur most frequently in the tongue. Other tumors that can occur are malignant lymphoid neoplasms, rhabdomyosarcomas and granular cell tumors. Most squamous cell carcinomas arise on the lateral side of the anterior two-thirds of tongue while it's rare on the dorsum of the tongue (Figure 11.3).

The musculature of the tongue provides a large volume of soft tissue for spread of the tumors. Infiltration of tumors tends to radiate from the initial focus in centrifugal manner within the muscle without any barrier. Infiltration usually proceeds in a backward direction. There is restriction of muscle movements when infiltration reaches the hyoglossus muscle. Tumors of the posterior third of the tongue are usually advanced when they involve the vallecula and epiglottis.

Tongue carcinomas metastasize to neck nodes early because of their rich lymphatic supply. Tumors of the anterior two-thirds of the tongue drain in Level IB and then to Level II while tumors from the posterior one-third of the tongue drain directly to Level II nodes. There can be skip metastasis to Level IV lymph nodes and is most commonly seen in tongue cancers (Lindberg et al.)[1].

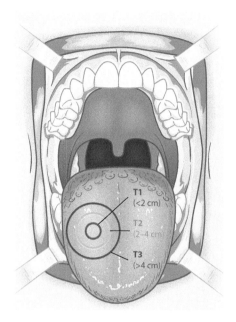
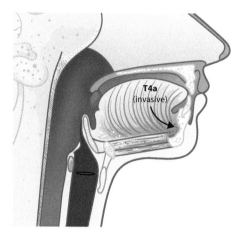

FIGURE 11.3   Carcinoma of tongue.

Tumors not crossing midline

1. *Wide glossectomy*: Tumors less than 2 cm
2. *Partial glossectomy*: Tumors less than 4 cm

Tumors crossing midline

1. *Hemi-glossectomy*: Tumors nearing midline of tongue
2. *Total glossectomy*: Tumors involving majority of tongue or midline lesions

Management

Management of the neck depends upon the N staging. Tumors of the tongue reaching FOM or tumors reaching the anterior tonsillar pillar can be approached by mandibular mandibulotomy and swing approach/pull through approach.

Reconstructive options

1. Primary closure
2. Tongue rotation and closure
3. *Regional flap*: Pectoralis major myocutaneous flap/submental flap
4. *Distant flap*: Free radial artery forearm flap/anterolateral thigh flap

Carcinoma of the Alveolus

Squamous cell carcinomas most commonly occur in the lower alveolus region when compared to the upper alveolus. Sometimes sarcomas can also occur here. Spread in the mandible is based on the presence or absence of teeth (Figure 11.4).

   Mandible with teeth: Periosteum is a strong hindrance to the spread of carcinomas in the mandible. The mucoperiosteal layer over the mylohyoid muscle is extensive, and hence, considerable time is taken for the spread of cancers. Teeth also protect as a barrier to prevent marginal spread

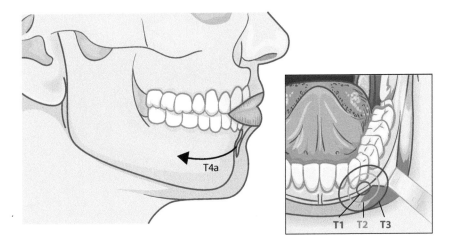

FIGURE 11.4 Carcinoma of the alveolus.

for lingual to buccal bone. Tumors advanced from the attached gingiva toward alveolus mostly in posterior molar region where the mylohyoid muscle is above the roots to the tooth, and the cancer advances through the dental sockets and then in to the cancellous bone of the mandible[1].

Mandible without teeth: There is resorption of the mandible with the loss of teeth, which brings the mylohyoid muscle close to the alveolar ridge. There is no barrier and the bone has small multiple foraminas on the alveolar ridge below the mucosa. Hence, it is an easy access for the carcinoma to spread to alveolar ridges, and then it enters into the medullary bone of the mandible.

Metastasis is to Level IB and then to Level II nodes.

Management

- *Tumor adjacent to but not fixed to the mandible*: Inner table of the periosteum to be removed
- *Tumor fixed to the periosteum*: Marginal mandibulectomy
- *Bony infiltration*: Segmental resection or hemimandibulectomy

Reconstructive options

1. No reconstruction
2. Reconstruction plate only
3. *Soft tissue*: Pectoralis major myocutaneous flap
4. *Bone tissue*: Fibula myocutaneous free flap

Carcinoma of the Retromolar Trigone

Squamous cell carcinomas arise most commonly in the retromolar trigone. As the anatomy of RMT is very restricted, tumors tend to spread quickly involving adjoining territories such as the buccal mucosa, soft palate, anterior tonsillar pillar, upper and lower alveoli and FOM. Medial spread of RMT cancers is more common than lateral spread.

The structure that is involved first in RMT cancers is the mandible deep to the trigone. This cancer can then reach the mandibular canal and can lead to perineural spread in proximal direction. Muscles first involved are the buccinator-pharyngeal complex on each side of pterygomandibular raphae, and beyond these infiltrated muscles are temporales that are attached to the ramus of the mandible. Infiltration of the bone commences from anterior segment and extends backward. The anterior segment is area of medullary

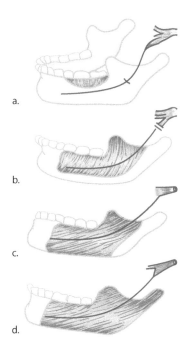

FIGURE 11.5   Layered resection of mandible for lesions approaching mandible and RMT lesions: (a) Alveolectomy, (b) marginal mandibulectomy, (c) segmental resection, (d) hemimandibulectomy.

bone immediately underlying the trigone, and the posterior end of trigone has the mandibular canal with its contents of nerve and then the coronoid process. The posterior most segment is the condylar segment[2].

Metastasis usually occurs in Level II nodes and occasionally in Level IB nodes.

Management

Mandibular resection in carcinoma of RMT is based on involvement of the mandible, with addition of resection of the inferior alveolar nerve at its point of exit from the foramen ovale if its involvement is suspected.

Layered resection of mandible (Figure 11.5)

• *Marginal mandibulectomy*: Removal of buccal and lingual cortical plates.
• *In-continuity resection with coronoid process*: In cases where inferior alveolar nerve and ascending ramus are involved by the tumor.
• *Segmental resection of mandible with sparing of condylar segment*
• *Arch sparing hemimandibulectomy*

Reconstruction (based on the size of the defect):

1. Split skin graft with buccal fat pad
2. *Local flaps*: Masseter muscle flap/forehead flap
3. *Regional flaps*: Pectoralis major myocutaneous flap/submental flap
4. *Distant flaps*: Radial artery forearm flap/fibula bone free flap/DCIA iliac free flap

Carcinoma of the Floor of Mouth

Virtually all tumors arising in the FOM are squamous cell carcinomas. This carcinoma can arise at any point in FOM. The floor can be divided into anterior and lateral FOM. The anterior part of FOM near the symphysis is most common, and resection of these tumors extending both sides of the sagittal plane is done.

Tumors of lateral FOM become deeply infiltrated and involve the sublingual gland anteriorly, the submandibular gland posteriorly, tongue medially and mandible laterally. Tumor spread in the tongue occurs vertical rather than horizontal, and hence, fixation of the tongue is seen to FOM causing ankyloglossia.

Metastasis of anterior FOM is to Level IA and then to Level IB lymph nodes while lateral FOM drains to Level IB nodes and then to Level II nodes.

Management

Anterior FOM

1. *Tumor adjacent to mandible but not fixed*: Resection of tumor and lingual cortex of the mandible
2. *Tumor fixed to periosteum*: Resection of tumor with marginal mandibulectomy
3. *Tumor involving mandible*: Anterior segmental resection (Andy Gump deformity)

Lateral FOM

Access is by lower lip splitting and mandibulotomy.

1. *Upper alveolectomy*: When tumor involves the alveolar portion of the mandible
2. *Rim resection*: When tumor involves the whole inner cortex
3. *Marginal mandibulectomy*: Tumor involving the upper end of the mandible but not invading it
4. *Segmental resection*: Tumors invading the mandible

Carcinoma of the Palate

Palatal squamous cell carcinomas often have a warty appearance. The tumor spreads marginally in a basically centrifugal manner but the significance of various directions of marginal spread varies, at least as far as the difficulty of resection and reconstruction is concerned. Spread occurs backward and forward along the lower ridge in the direction of the molar region and the incisor region, medially toward the center of the palate, laterally toward the upper buccal sulcus. If the initial site is on the palatal side, it spreads to occur mainly toward the center of the palate; if the initial site is on buccal side, spread is more toward the upper buccal sulcus. Deep spread of the tumor involves the bone immediately underlying the mucosa. The speed with which the bone is penetrated and the antral or nasal mucosa involved depends very much on the thickness of the bone locally, and this varies considerably in different sites[1,2].

Carcinoma of the Soft Palate

Squamous cell carcinoma arising on the soft palate is extremely rare. When the tumor remains confined to the depth of the soft palate, spread merely brings the tumor to its nasal surface. From a resection point of view, it is, consequently, a marginal spread, which has to be considered. This can carry tumor on to the hard palate, though spread in this longitudinal direction rarely occurs. Most important is spread laterally on anterior faucial pillars.

Lymph node metastasis from a primary tumor confined to the hard palate is not very common. Spread from the soft palate can occur in upper deep jugular lymph nodes[2].

Management: Hard palate and upper alveolus

Excision: Monobloc resection/layered resection of the object is to resect the complete tumor as a single block of tissue. The assumption is made at the outset that the underlying bone is involved by tumor and must be excised along with the mucoperiosteum that overlies it. Once the soft tissue has been isolated by the initial encircling incision, an osteotome with a mallet is used to divide the bone underlying the mucoperiosteum in the same circumferential line (Figure 11.6).

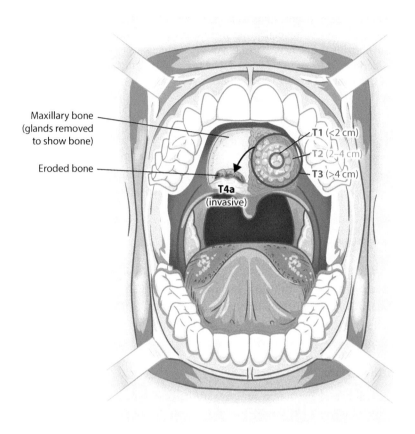

Maxillary bone
(glands removed
to show bone)

Eroded bone

T4a
(invasive)

T1 (<2 cm)
T2 (2–4 cm)
T3 (>4 cm)

FIGURE 11.6 Carcinoma of the palate.

Layered resection: Instead of a single-block resection, the tumor is removed in layers: First, the
oral mucoperiosteum is removed, next the underlying bone, and last, if necessary, the antral
and/or nasal mucoperiosteum is removed.

Reconstruction

1. Secondary intention healing without reconstruction
2. Split skin grafting
3. Local flaps such as palatal flaps/tongue flaps

Carcinomas Extending to the Infratemporal Fossa (ITF)

Locally advanced oral cavity cancers such as buccal mucosa, retromolar trigone cancers, lower alveolus
extending to infratemporal fossa (ITF) pose a great challenge to head and neck surgeons. According
to AJCC/UICC, these tumors are classified as T4b lesions; the tumor extends to MS, pterygoid muscles (PM) and PP. Lately, these tumors were once considered unresectable lesions and treated pallia-
tively. From a very few years, numerous studies have published in the literature that these tumors can be
resected with a reasonably favorable prognosis by compartment resection of ITF, particularly when the
tumor was below sigmoid notch of mandible. Some studies advise to downstage the tumor by neoadjuvant chemotherapy and then evaluate and proceed with the surgical plan and then adjuvant concurrent

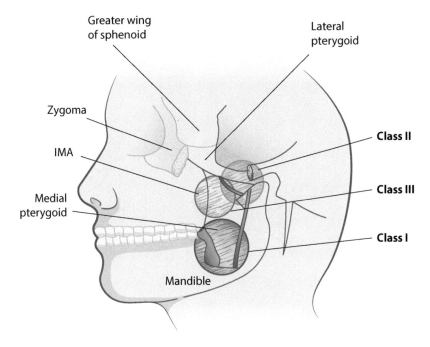

Zygoma

IMA

Greater wing
of sphenoid

Lateral
pterygoid

Medial
pterygoid

Class II

Class III

Class I

Mandible

FIGURE 11.7 Classification of ITF.

chemoradiation. Close margins of resection, extra nodal spread from lymph nodes and supra notch and involvement of posterior part of ITF were factors which predisposed to recurrence. Recently, ITF tumors have been classified based on the anatomical structures involved[3] (Figure 11.7).

Management Protocol NCCN Clinical Practice Guidelines in Oncology (NCCN Guidelines) for Head and Neck Cancers V.2.2019 for Oral Cavity Cancers[4]

Depending on the evidence, NCCN consensus for these recommendations may vary.

If T1-2, N0:

a. Resection of primary tumor (preferred) with/without ipsilateral or bilateral neck dissection. **(or)**

b. Resection of primary with/without sentinel lymph node biopsy. If SLN identification is successful then and if it's N0, follow-up is required. If it's N+ then perform neck dissection. **(or)**

c. Definitive radiation. If no residual disease radiation then follow-up of patient. If there is residual disease then perform salvage surgery.

After doing a, b, or c, if there is one positive node, consider adjuvant radiation. If there is extracapsular spread, prefer adjuvant chemoradiation. If there positive margin then prefer re-resection or RT or chemoradiation.

If T3N0, T1-3 N1-3, T4a Any N:

d. *Surgery*:

1. *N0, N1, N2a-b, N3*: Resection of primary, ipsilateral or bilateral neck dissection

2. *N2c*: Resection of primary and bilateral neck dissection

After performing 1 or 2, if there is no extracapsular spread or positive margins then radiation is optional. Chemoradiation is the preferred treatment for extranodal extension. If in positive margin, go for re-resection or RT or chemoradiation.

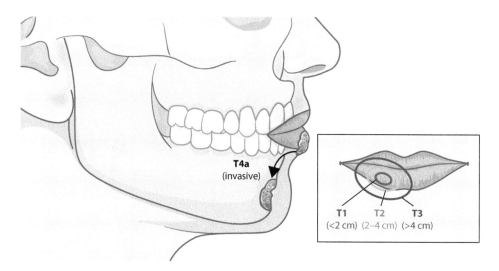

FIGURE 11.8   Carcinoma of the lip.

• *Mutimodality clinical trials*

Carcinoma of the Lip:

Lips form the anterior boundary of the oral cavity that is lined by non-stratified squamous epithelium. The mucosa of the lips covers the orbicularis oris muscle underneath with a distance of only 2 mm. Therefore, any ulcerative lesion on lips gets fixed quite early. The incidence of cancer of lower lip is 93%, upper lip is 5% and commissure is only 2%. The upper lip and lower lips has a cutaneous lymphatic spread. In lower lip, there are two collecting lymphatic ducts—medial duct draining the inner layer of lip and lateral duct draining the lateral side of both the outer-third of lower lips. Drainage of the upper lip is to preauricular, infraparotid, submandibular, and submental lymph nodes (Figure 11.8).

Management options

1. Lip shave
2. Wedge excision

Reconstruction options

Refer to *Surgeon's Knife: Head and Neck Incisions by Akheel Mohammad, Jaypee Medical Publishers, 2016.*

1. *Lower lip*:
   a. *Less than one-third*: Primary closure
   b. *One-third to two-thirds*: Abbe, Abbe-Estlander, or Karapandzic flap
   c. *>Two-thirds*: Bilateral Gillies fan flaps, axial scalp flap or free tissue transfer
2. *Upper lip*:
   a. *Less than one-third*: Primary closure or Abbe flap
   b. *One-third to two-thirds*: Reverse Karapandzic flap or peri-alar advancement
   c. *>Two-thirds*: Reverse Karapandzic or Abbe flap, combination peri-alar advancement,
   d. Rarely bilateral nasolabial flaps, Gilies fan flaps or free tissue transfer
3. *Commissure*:
   a. Abbe-Estlander, double rhomboid flaps or free tissue transfer

Management Protocol NCCN Guidelines for Head and Neck Cancers V.2.2019 for Lip Cancers

Depending on the evidence, NCCN consensus for these recommendations may vary.

4. *If T1-2, N0:*
   a. Surgical resection is preferred, but elective neck dissection is not recommended. If there is positive margins then go for re-resection or radiation. **(or)**
   b. Perform definitive radiation on the primary site. If there is residual or recurrent tumor post radiation then go for surgical resection and reconstruction.

5. *If T3, T4a, N0 or Any T, N1-3:*
   1. *Surgery:*
      a. *N0:* Resection of primary with/without ipsilateral or bilateral neck dissection.
      b. *N1, N2a-b, N3:* Resection of primary, ipsilateral neck dissection with/without contralateral neck dissection.
      c. *N2c:* Resection of primary and bilateral neck dissection.

      After performing a, b, or c, if there is one positive node with no extracapsular spread then refer the patient for radiation. If there is extracapsular spread then refer for chemoradiation or radiation. If positive margins are seen then re-resection may be done.

      (or)
   2. *Definitive radiation or chemoradiation:*
      a. Obtain complete clinical response of the primary site (N0 at initial staging) then follow up the patient periodically.
      b. Obtain complete clinical response of the primary site (N+ at initial staging). If there is residual tumor in the neck, perform neck dissection after radiation/chemoradiation. If complete response of the neck is performed then follow up the patient.
      c. If there is less response of primary site after radiation/chemoradiation then perform salvage surgery + neck dissection.

REFERENCES

1. Watkinson J, Gilbert R. *Stell & Maran's textbook of head and neck surgery and oncology.* CRC Press; 2011 Dec 30.
2. McGregor IA, McGregor FM. *Cancer of the face and mouth: pathology and management for surgeons.* Churchill Livingstone; 1986.
3. Trivedi NP, Kekatpure V, Kuriakose MA. Radical (compartment) resection for advanced buccal cancer involving masticator space (T4b): our experience in thirty patients. *Clinical Otolaryngology.* 2012 Dec;37(6):477–83.
4. Referenced with permission from the NCCN Guidelines® for Head and Neck Cancers V.2.2019 © National Comprehensive Cancer Network, Inc. 2019. All rights reserved. Accessed [July 12, 2019] *Available online at* www.NCCN.org. NCCN makes no warranties of any kind whatsoever regarding their content, use or application and disclaims any responsibility for their application or use in any way.

12

Pharynx

Pharynx Tumors[1]

- **Primary site**
  - *Nasopharynx*: Anterior at posterior choana along the plane of airway to the level of free border of soft palate.
  - *Pharyngeal involvement*: Posterolateral infiltration of tumor extending beyond the pharyngobasilar fascia.
  - *Masticatory involvement*: Tumor extending beyond the anterior surface of lateral pterygoid muscle or tumor extending to posterolateral wall of maxillary antrum and pterygomaxillary fissure.
  - *Oropharynx*: From plane of superior surface of soft palate to hyoid bone.
  - *Hypopharynx*: From the plane of super surface of hyoid bone to lower border of the cricoid cartilage.
- **Regional lymph nodes**
  - *Very high spread.*
  - *Nasopharynx*: Retropharyngeal, upper-jugular (level II) lymph nodes.
  - *Oropharynx*: Upper and mid-jugular (level III) lymph nodes.
  - *Hypopharynx*: Para-pharyngeal, tracheal, and mid and lower jugular (level IV) lymph nodes.
  - Bilateral drainage is common in pharyngeal tumors.
- **Clinical staging**
  - Based on inspection + direct or indirect endoscopy.
  - *Studies included*: MRI and CT scans.
  - *Complete endoscopy*: Assess surface extent and perform biopsy.

TNM Classification

Nasopharynx (Figure 12.1)

- *T1*: Confined only to the nasopharynx
- *T2*: Extends to soft tissues
- *T2a*: Extends to the oropharynx and nasal cavity without parapharyngeal extension
- *T2b*: Any tumor with parapharyngeal extension
- *T3*: Involves bony structures and paranasal sinuses
- *T4*: Intracranial extension and involvement of cranial nerves, infratemporal fossa, hypopharynx, orbit, or masticator space

DOI: 10.1201/9780367822019-12

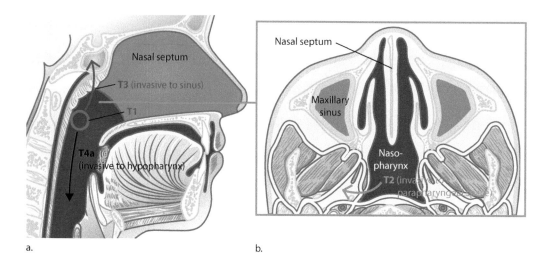

FIGURE 12.1   Carcinoma of nasopharynx: (a) sagittal section, (b) axial section.

Regional lymph nodes
- *NX*: Cannot be assessed
- *N0*: No regional lymph node metastasis
- *N1*: Unilateral metastasis is 6 cm or less in diameter, above the supraclavicular fossa
- *N2*: Bilateral metastasis is 6 cm or less in diameter, above the supraclavicular fossa
- *N3*: Metastasis is >6 cm and to supraclavicular fossa
- *N3a*: It is >6 cm in diameter
- *N3b*: Extension to the supraclavicular fossa

Staging for nasopharynx
- *Stage 0*: Tis N0 M0
- *Stage I*: T1 N0 M0
- *Stage IIA*: T2a N0 M0
- *Stage IIB*: T1 N1 M0
    - T2 N1 M0
    - T2a N1 M0
    - T2b N0 M0
    - T2b N1 M0
- *Stage III*: T1 N2 M0
    - T2a N2 M0
    - T2b N2 M0
    - T3 N0 M0
    - T3 N1 M0
    - T3 N2 M0
- *Stage IVA*: T4 N0 M0
    - T4 N1 M0
    - T4 N2 M0
- *Stage IVB*: Any T N3 M0
- *Stage IVC*: Any T, any N M1

Management Protocol NCCN Clinical Practice Guidelines in Oncology (NCCN Guidelines) for Head and Neck Cancers V.2.2019 for Nasopharynx Cancers[2]

Depending on the evidence, the NCCN consensus for these recommendations may vary.

1. *If T1N0M0*:

   Definitive radiation to nasopharynx and elective radiation to neck

2. *If T1N1-3, T2-4, any N*:

   a. Concurrent chemoradiation followed by adjuvant chemotherapy (**or**)

   b. Concurrent chemoradiation not followed by adjuvant chemotherapy (**or**)

   c. Induction chemotherapy followed by chemoradiation

   After point a, b, or c, if there is a residual tumor in the neck, perform neck dissection. If there is a complete clinical response, observe.

3. *Any T, any N, M1*:

   RT alone or surgery are also options for select patients with oligometastatic disease.

   a. Platinum-based combination chemotherapy

   b. Concurrent chemoradiation

Oropharynx

- *T1*: 2 cm or less in diameter
- *T2*: > 2 cm but < 4 cm in diameter
- *T3*: > 4 cm in diameter
- *T4a*: Invades the larynx, deep/extrinsic muscle of tongue, medial pterygoid, hard palate, or mandible
- *T4b*: Invades lateral pterygoid muscle, pterygoid plates, lateral nasopharynx, or skull base or encases carotid artery

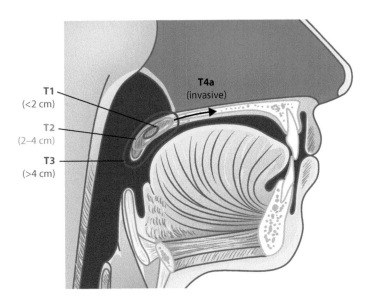

FIGURE 12.2   Carcinoma of oropharynx (Sagittal section).

Management Protocol NCCN Guidelines® for Head and Neck Cancers V.2.2019 for Oropharynx Cancers (Figure 12.2)[2]

Depending on the evidence, the NCCN consensus for these recommendations may vary.

For p16-negative disease:

1. *If T1-2,N0-1*:
   a. *Definitive radiation*: If there is a complete response, follow up. If there is a residual disease after radiation, perform salvage surgery **(or)**
   b. Transoral or open resection of primary with ipsilateral or bilateral neck dissection. If there is extracapsular spread, give chemoradiation. If there is a positive margin, perform re-resection if feasible **(or)**
   c. For T2, N1 only, radiation + systemic chemotherapy. If complete a response, follow up or if there is a residual disease, perform salvage surgery **(or)**
   d. Multimodality clinical trials
2. *If T3-4a, N0-1*:
   a. Concurrent systemic therapy/radiation. If no complete response, perform salvage surgery **(or)**
   b. Transoral or open resection for primary and neck. If there is extracapsular spread and/or positive margin, follow adjuvant chemoradiation **(or)**
   c. Induction chemotherapy followed by radiation or chemoradiation. If there is a residual disease, perform salvage surgery **(or)**
   d. Multimodality clinical trials
3. *Any T, N2-3*:
   a. Concurrent systemic therapy/radiation **(or)**
   b. Induction chemotherapy followed by radiation or chemoradiation **(or)**
   c. After point (a) or (b), if the primary site shows complete response but a residual tumor in the neck, perform neck dissection. If the primary site shows residual tumor, perform salvage surgery and neck dissection
   d. *Transoral or open resection*: Primary and neck. After resection and ipsilateral/bilateral neck dissection if there is extracapsular spread/positive margin, give adjuvant chemoradiation **(or)**
   e. Multimodality clinical trials

Hypopharynx
   a. *T1*: Limited to 1 subsite of HP and 2 cm or < in diameter.
   b. *T2*: Invades > 1 subsite of HP or an adjacent site or measures > 2 cm but < 4 cm diameter without fixation of hemilarynx.
   c. *T3*: > 4 cm diameter or with fixation of hemilarynx.
   d. *T4a*: Invades thyroid/cricoid cartilage, hyoid bone, thyroid gland, esophagus, or central compartment soft tissue.
   e. *T4b*: Invades prevertebral fascia, encases carotid artery, or involves mediastinal structures.

Management Protocol NCCN Guidelines for Head and Neck Cancers V.2.2019 for Hypopharynx Cancers (Figure 12.3)[2]

Depending on the evidence, the NCCN consensus for these recommendations may vary.

Most T1 N0, selected T2 N0:

1. *Definitive radiation*: Residual tumor in primary site then performs salvage surgery with neck dissection. **(or)**

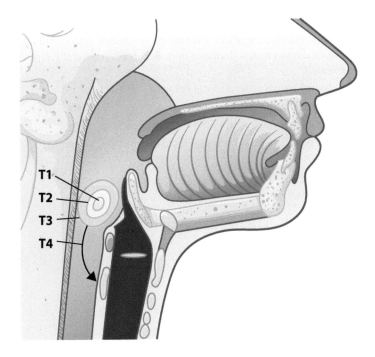

FIGURE 12.3 Carcinoma of hypopharynx (sagittal section) 2.

2. *Surgery*: Palatal laryngopharyngectomy with ipsilateral or bilateral neck dissection. If there is extra-capsular spread, give adjuvant chemoradiation. If there is a positive margin, perform re-resection

3. Multimodal clinical trials

T2-3, any N; T1, N+ if requiring pharyngectomy with total laryngectomy:

4. *Induction chemotherapy*: If there is a complete response, consider RT or chemoradiation. If there is partial response, consider surgery and then chemoradiation if any adverse effects **(or)**

5. *Laryngopharyngectomy with neck dissection, including level VI*: If there is extracapsular spread/positive margin, give adjuvant chemoradiation **(or)**

6. *Concurrent systemic therapy*: If there is a primary site complete response, follow-up with the patient but if there is residual in the neck, perform neck dissection. If residual is in the primary site, salvage surgery with neck dissection **(or)**

7. Multimodality clinical trials

If T4, any N:

8. Surgery with neck dissection preferred followed by adjuvant chemoradiation if extranodal extension and/or positive margin **(or)**

9. *Induction chemotherapy*: If there is complete response, go with radiation or chemoradiation. If there is below partial response, plan for surgery with neck and then chemoradiation **(or)**

10. Concurrent systemic therapy **(or)**

11. Multimodality clinical trial

Regional lymph nodes (for Oropharynx and Hypopharynx)

- *NX*: Cannot be assessed
- *N0*: No regional lymph node metastasis

- *N1*: Single ipsilateral lymph node is 3 cm or less in diameter
- *N2*: Single ipsilateral lymph node is >3 cm but <6 cm in greatest diameter or multiple ipsilateral lymph nodes are <6 cm in greatest diameter or in B/L or contralateral lymph nodes are <6 cm in greatest diameter
- *N2a*: Single ipsilateral lymph node is >3 cm but <6 cm in diameter
- *N2b*: Multiple ipsilateral lymph nodes are <6 cm in greatest diameter
- *N2c*: B/L or contralateral lymph nodes are <6 cm in diameter
- *N3*: Metastasis in a lymph node is more than 6 cm in greatest diameter

Distant metastasis(M):

- *MX*: Metastasis cannot be assessed
- *M0*: No distant metastasis
- *M1*: Distant metastasis

Staging for oropharynx and hypopharynx:

- *Stage 0*: Tis N0 M0
- *Stage I*: T1 N0 M0
- *Stage II*: T2 N0 M0
- *Stage III*: T3 N0 M0
  - T1 N1 M0
  - T2 N1 M0
  - T3 N1 M0
- *Stage IVA*: T4a N0 M0
  - T4a N1 M0
  - T1 N2 M0
  - T2 N2 M0
  - T3 N2 M0
  - T4a N2 M0
- *Stage IVB*: T4b any N M0
  - Any T N3 M0
- *Stage IVC*: Any T any N M1

REFERENCES

1. Watkinson J, Gilbert R. Stell & Maran's textbook of head and neck surgery and oncology. CRC Press; 2011 Dec 30.
2. Referenced with permission from the NCCN Guidelines for Head and Neck Cancers V.2.2019 © National Comprehensive Cancer Network, Inc. 2019. All rights reserved. Accessed [July and Day 12, 2019]. *Available online at*: http://www.NCCN.org. NCCN makes no warranties of any kind whatsoever regarding their content, use or application and disclaims any responsibility for their application or use in any way.

13

Larynx

Larynx

Primary site

- *Supraglottis*:
  - Suprahyoid epiglottis
  - Infrahyoid epiglottis
  - Aryepiglottic folds
  - Arytenoids
  - Ventricular bands (false cords)
- *Glottis*: True vocal cords
- *Subglottis*: Subglottis

Regional lymph nodes

- *True vocal cords*: Rarely spread to lymph nodes
- *Supraglottis*: Upper and mid jugular (Levels II, III)
- *Glottis*: Directly to adjacent soft tissues and pretracheal and paratracheal and laryngeal + upper, middle, and lower jugular nodes
- *Subglottis*: Contralateral spread to lymph nodes is common

Clinical staging:

- *Assessment*: Inspection + direct mirror and endoscopic examination with fiberoptic nasolaryngoscope
- *Tumor details*: Confirmed histologically and biopsies included
- *Cross-sectional imaging*: To find the extent of the primary tumor
- *Complete endoscopy*: To assess the primary tumor for documentation and perform tumor biopsy

TNM classification

Supraglottis (Figure 13.1)

- *T1*: Limited to one anatomic subsite of supraglottis with normal vocal cord mobility
- *T2*: Invades mucosa of more than one adjacent anatomic subsite of supraglottis or glottis or region outside the supraglottis (e.g., mucosa of base of tongue, vallecula, medial wall of pyriform sinus) without fixation of the larynx
- *T3*: Limited to larynx with vocal cord fixation and/or invades any of the following: postcricoid area, pre-epiglottic tissues
- *T4a*: Invades through the thyroid cartilage and/or invades tissues extending beyond larynx
- *T4b*: Invades that prevertebral space encases carotid artery or invades other mediastinal structures

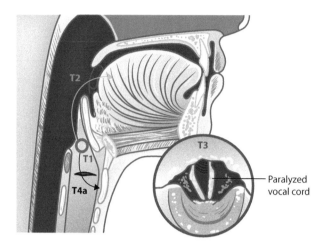

FIGURE 13.1 Carcinoma of supraglottis (sagittal section).

Management Protocol NCCN Clinical Practice Guidelines in Oncology (NCCN Guidelines) for Head and Neck Cancers V.2.2019 for Supraglottic Larynx Cancer[1]

Depending on the evidence, NCCN consensus for these recommendations may vary.

1. Amenable to larynx preserving (conservation surgery), most T1–T2, N0, selected T3 patients:
   a. Endoscopic resection with neck dissection (**or**)
   b. Open partial supraglottic laryngectomy with neck dissection (**or**)
   c. After point (a) or (b), if it's T1–T2, N0, then follow up the patient. If found one positive node, consider adjuvant radiation. If found positive node with positive margins, consider re-resection or radiation or chemoradiation. If there is extracapsular spread, then consider chemoradiation.
   d. Definitive radiation

   After performing 4– to 8– week clinical assessment, if there is partial response or metastasis, perform a CT scan/PET-CT scan. If no metastasis diagnosis is confirmed, perform surgery with neck dissection.

2. Requiring (amenable to) total laryngectomy (T3, N0):
   a. *Concurrent systemic therapy/radiation*: If there is a complete response in the primary site, follow up the patient. If there is residual tumor, perform salvage surgery with neck dissection (**or**)
   b. *Laryngectomy ipsilateral thyroidectomy with ipsilateral or bilateral neck dissection*: If found N0 or one positive node, consider adjuvant radiation. If there is extracapsular spread/positive margin, consider adjuvant chemoradiation (**or**)
   c. Go for radiation if patient is not medical candidate for concurrent systemic therapy/radiation (**or**)
   d. *Induction chemotherapy*: If there is a complete response, go for radiation. If there is no response, go for systemic chemotherapy/RT. If partial response, go for RT or chemoradiation; if less than partial, follow surgery or treatment based on performance status (**or**).
   e. Multimodality clinical trials

3. Amenable to larynx preserving (conservation) surgery, *T1–T2, N+ and selected T3, N1*:
   a. Concurrent systemic therapy/radiation (**or**)
   b. Definitive radiation for low-volume disease or for patients who are medically unfit for concurrent systemic therapy/RT (**or**)

After point (a) or (b), if there is complete clinical response in primary tumor and residual in the neck, perform neck dissection. If there is residual in primary side, perform salvage surgery with neck dissection.

   c. *Partial supraglottic laryngectomy and neck dissection*: If there is extracapsular spread/positive margin, consider adjuvant chemoradiation **(or)**

   d. *Induction chemotherapy*: If there is a complete response, go for radiation. If there is no response, go for systemic chemotherapy/RT. If partial response, go for RT or chemoradiation; if less than partial, then follow surgery or treatment based on performance status **(or)**

   e. Multimodality clinical trials

4. Requiring (amenable to) total laryngectomy, (most T3, N2–N3):

   a. *Concurrent systemic therapy/radiation*: If primary site complete response and residual tumor in the neck then perform neck dissection. If there is a residual tumor in the primary site, perform salvage surgery with neck dissection **(or)**

   b. Laryngectomy, ipsilateral thyroidectomy with neck dissection. If there are extracapsular spread and positive margin, perform adjuvant chemoradiation **(or)**

   c. *Induction chemotherapy*: If there is a complete response, go for radiation. If there is no response, go for systemic chemotherapy/RT. If partial response, go for RT or chemoradiation; if less than partial, follow surgery or treatment based on performance status **(or)**

   d. Multimodality clinical trials

5. *If T4a, N0–N3*: Laryngectomy, thyroidectomy with ipsilateral or bilateral neck dissection. If there is extracapsular spread/positive margin, give adjuvant chemoradiation.

6. *If T4a, N0–N3 patients who decline surgery:*

   a. Consider concurrent chemoradiation. If primary site complete response but tumor is in the neck, perform neck dissection, if residual in primary site, perform salvage surgery with neck dissection **(or)**

   b. Clinical trial **(or)**

   c. *Induction chemotherapy*: If there is a complete response, go for radiation. If there is no response, go for systemic chemotherapy/RT. If partial response, go for RT or chemoradiation; if less than partial, follow surgery or treatment based on performance status

Glottis (Figure 13.2)

   o *T1*: Limited to vocal cord(s) which may involve anterior or posterior commissure with normal mobility.

   o *T1a*: Limited to only one vocal cord.

   o *T1b*: Involves both the vocal cords.

   o *T2*: Extends to supraglottis and/or subglottis, and/or with impaired vocal cord mobility

   o *T3*: Limited to the larynx with fixation of vocal cord.

   o *T4a*: Invades through the thyroid cartilage and/or invades tissues beyond the larynx (e.g., soft tissues of the neck, trachea, including deep intrinsic muscles of tongue, strap muscles, thyroid, or esophagus).

   o *T4b*: Invades that prevertebral space may encase carotid artery or invades mediastinal structures.

Management Protocol NCCN Clinical Practice Guidelines in Oncology (NCCN Guidelines) for Head and Neck Cancers V.2.2019 for Glottic Larynx Cancers[1]

Depending on the evidence, NCCN consensus for these recommendations may vary.

7. *Carcinoma in situ*: Endoscopic resection (preferred) **(or)** radiation.

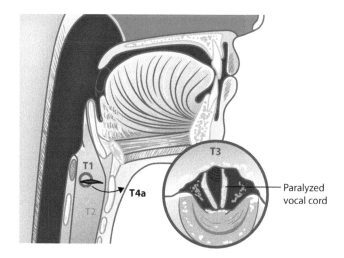

FIGURE 13.2   Carcinoma of the glottis.

8. *Amenable to larynx-preserving (conservation) surgery (**T1–T2 or select T3**)*: Radiation **(or)** partial laryngectomy/endoscopic or open resection. If there is extracapsular spread, give chemoradiation. If there is positive margin, perform re-resection or radiation.

9. T3 requiring (amenable to total laryngectomy) **(N0–N1)**:

   a. *Concurrent systemic therapy/radiation*: If primary site shows complete clinical response (N0 at initial staging), follow-up of the patient is required. If there is complete clinical response of the primary site but residual tumor in the neck, perform neck dissection. If there is a residual tumor in primary site, perform salvage surgery with neck dissection **(or)**

   b. *Surgery*: If N0 neck, perform laryngectomy with ipsilateral thyroidectomy. If N1 neck, perform laryngectomy with ipsilateral thyroidectomy, ipsilateral neck dissection, or bilateral neck dissection. If there is extracapsular spread/positive margin, give chemoradiation **(or)**

   c. Induction chemotherapy **(or)**

   d. Multimodality clinical trials

10. T3 requiring (amenable to) total laryngectomy **(N2–N3)**:

    a. *Concurrent systemic therapy/radiation*: If primary site shows a complete response with a residual tumor in the neck after this initial treatment, perform neck dissection. If there is a residual primary tumor, perform salvage surgery with neck dissection **(or)**

    b. *Surgery*: Laryngectomy with ipsilateral thyroidectomy, ipsilateral or bilateral neck dissection. If there is extracapsular spread and/or positive margin, give chemoradiation **(or)**.

    c. Induction chemotherapy **(or)**

    d. Multimodality clinical trials

11. ***T4a, Any N***:

    a. *Surgery*: If N0 neck, perform total laryngectomy with thyroidectomy with/without unilateral or bilateral neck dissection. If N1 neck, perform total laryngectomy with thyroidectomy, ipsilateral neck dissection with/without contralateral neck dissection. If N2–N3, perform total laryngectomy with thyroidectomy, ipsilateral, or bilateral neck dissection.

    After performing surgery, consider adjuvant radiation or chemoradiation or observation for highly selected patients.

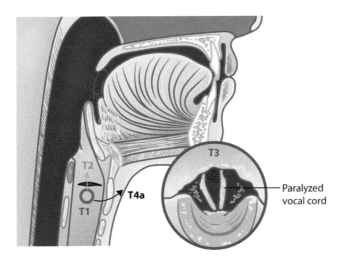

FIGURE 13.3 Carcinoma of the subglottis (sagittal section).

12. Selected T4a patients who decline surgery:
    a. *Consider concurrent chemoradiation*: If primary site shows a complete response but tumor is in the neck, perform neck dissection. If residual in primary site, perform salvage surgery with neck dissection **(or)**
    b. Clinical trial for function preserving surgical or nonsurgical management **(or)**
    c. Induction chemotherapy

Subglottis (Figure 13.3)

- *T1*: Limited to the subglottis
- *T2*: Extends to one or both vocal cord(s) with normal or impaired mobility
- *T3*: Limited to larynx with vocal cord fixation
- *T4a*: Invades the cricoid or thyroid cartilage and/or invades tissues beyond the larynx (e.g., soft tissues of the neck, trachea, including deep intrinsic muscles of tongue, strap muscles, thyroid, or esophagus)
- *T4b*: Invades prevertebral space may encase carotid artery or invades mediastinal structures

Regional lymph nodes (N)
- *NX*: It cannot be assessed
- *N0*: No regional lymph node metastasis
- *N1*: Single ipsilateral lymph node is 3 cm or less in diameter
- *N2*: Single ipsilateral lymph node is >3 cm but <6 cm in diameter or in multiple ipsilateral lymph nodes, <6 cm in diameter or in b/l or contralateral lymph nodes <6 cm in diameter
- *N2a*: Single ipsilateral lymph node is >3 cm but <6 cm in diameter
- *N2b*: Multiple ipsilateral lymph nodes are <6 cm in diameter
- *N2c*: Bilateral or contralateral lymph nodes are <6 cm in diameter
- *N3*: Lymph node is >6 cm in greatest diameter.

Distant metastasis (M)
- *MX*: Metastasis cannot be assessed
- M0: No distant metastasis
- *M1*: Distant metastasis

Staging for larynx

- *Stage 0*: Tis N0 M0
- *Stage I*: T1 N0 M0
- *Stage II*: T2 N0 M0
- *Stage III*: T3 N0 M0
    - T1 N1 M0
    - T2 N1 M0
    - T3 N1 M0
- *Stage IVA*: T4a N0 M0
    - T4a N1 M0
    - Any T N2 M0
- Stage IVB: T4b Any N M0
    - Any T N3 M0
- *Stage IVC*: Any T, Any N M1

REFERENCE

1. Referenced with permission from the NCCN Guidelines for Head and Neck Cancers V.2.2019 © National Comprehensive Cancer Network, Inc. 2019. All rights reserved. Accessed [July and Day 12, 2019]. *Available online at*: http://www.NCCN.org . NCCN makes no warranties of any kind whatsoever regarding their content, use or application and disclaims any responsibility for their application or use in any way.

14

Paranasal Sinuses

Paranasal Sinus

Primary sites
- *Maxillary sinus*: Most common of sinonasal malignancies
- *Ethmoidal sinus*: Less common

Regional lymph nodes
- Mostly uncommon
- Advanced maxillary sinus cancers spread to buccinator muscle, submandibular, jugular lymph nodes
- Ethmoidal sinus cancers are prone less for lymphatic spread
- *Advanced primary cancers*: Bilateral lymphatic spread may occur

Clinical staging
- *Assessment*: Nasal endoscopy with rigid or flexible fiberoptic instrument is recommended
- *MRI or CT scan*: More accurate for pretreatment staging

Carcinoma of Maxillary Sinuses

Carcinoma of the maxillary antrum is rarely diagnosed as it is still confined within the antrum. The mode of clinical presentation is determined by which surface of the antrum is infiltrated and where the surrounding structures tumor appears. Extension appears generally in one direction, though occasionally more than one involved from the outset. The tumor foci within the antrum, even though the mass of tumor, may also have expanded in polypoidal manner to fill the antral cavity. Extension out with the antrum can occur in five main directions. There can be loose dentition, ulceration in the alveolar region extending downwards, toward the oral cavity, and is the first sign of subperiosteal swelling in the vicinity of alveolar ridge near the upper buccal sulcus. It can extend anteriorly in to the cheek and produces diffuse bulge, obliterating in nasolabial fold and creating facial asymmetry. It can extend upwards through the antral roof/orbital floor, into the orbit. The most frequent site is anterior and swelling of the infraorbital margin is produced, palpable behind the lower eyelid. It can extend medially into the nasal cavity and gives rise to nasal discharge, clear and watery, purulent or blood-stained. Small repeated epistaxis may occur. It can extend backwards in direction of the pterygoid plates and the muscles of the pterygoid fossa. This type of extension tends to be silent until it is very advanced involving the maxillary division of the trigeminal and other nerves in the area. In addition to these modes of spread, extension can take place into ethmoids also[1].

TNM Classification

Maxillary Sinuses (Figure 14.1)
- *T1*: Tumors limited to mucosa of maxillary sinus with no erosion or destruction of bone
- *T2*: Causing erosion of bone or destruction with extension to hard palate and/or the middle of the nasal meatus, except the extension to the posterior wall of maxillary sinus and pterygoid plates

Tumors of the Maxillary Sinus

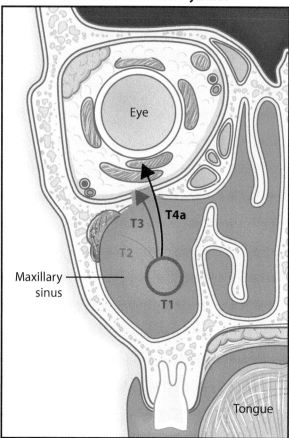

FIGURE 14.1   Carcinoma of maxillary sinus (coronal section).

- *T3*: Invades any of the following: bone of the posterior wall of maxillary sinus, subcutaneous tissues, floor or medial wall of orbit, pterygoid fossa, ethmoid sinuses.
- *T4a*: Invades anterior orbital contents, pterygoid plates, skin of cheek, infratemporal fossa, cribriform plate, sphenoid or frontal sinuses
- *T4b*: Invades any of the following: orbital apex, dura, brain, middle cranial fossa, cranial nerves other than maxillary division of trigeminal nerve (V_2), nasopharynx, or clivus

Ohngren's Line (Figure 14.2)
It is an imaginary line drawn from angle of mandible to medial canthus of eye.
- *Anterior (Inferior) to the line*: Benign tumors
- *Posterior (Superior) to the line*: Malignant tumors[2]

Management options
1. *Partial maxillectomy*: Lesions involving lower part of alveolus and maxillary sinus
2. *Subtotal maxillectomy*: Lesions involving more than half of the maxillary sinus
3. *Total maxillectomy*: Lesions involving complete maxillary sinus
4. *Total maxillectomy with orbital eccenteration*: Lesions of maxillary sinus involving orbit

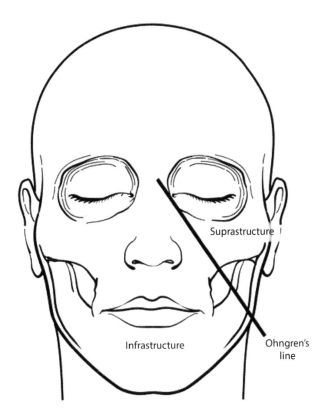

FIGURE 14.2 Ohngren's line.

Management Protocol NCCN Clinical Practice Guidelines in Oncology (NCCN Guidelines) for Head and Neck Cancers V.2.2019 for Maxillary Sinus Cancers[3]

Depending on the evidence, the NCCN consensus for these recommendations may vary.

1. *T1–T2, N0 All histologies except adenoid cystic*: Perform surgical resection. If the margins negative, then follow up the patient. If there is perineural invasion, then consider adjuvant radiation or chemoradiation. If there is positive margin, then perform surgical re-resection if possible
2. *If T1–T2, N0 adenoid cystic*: Perform surgical resection and adjuvant RT is recommended for these patients
3. *If T3–T4a, N0*: Complete surgical resection: If there is extracapsular spread/positive margin, then give adjuvant radiation or chemoradiation
4. *If T4b, any N*: Clinical trial **(or)** definitive radiation **(or)** chemoradiation
5. *If T1–T4a, N+*: Surgical resection with neck dissection. If there is extracapsular spread, then adjuvant radiation or consider chemoradiation

Nasal Cavity and Ethmoidal Sinuses

Ethmoidal and labyrinth tumors indicate their presence clinically because of the direction of extension (Figure 14.3). If this is predominantly lateral, it can cause dislocation of the eyeball and diplopia with the development of a diffuse indurated swelling in inner canthal area if the anterior cells are predominantly involved. In the process of extending laterally, the periorbita is unexpectedly effective as a barrier to spread into the orbit, though it is one which is of course ultimately breached[2].

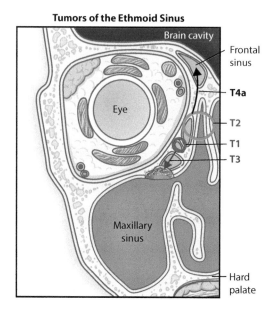

FIGURE 14.3 Carcinoma of ethmoid sinus (coronal section).

Lymph node metastasis is to upper deep jugular chain. Treatment of maxillary tumors and ethmoidal tumors is, respectively, maxillectomy and ethmoidectomy with or without maxillectomy. If orbit is involved, orbital exenteration is referred.

Reconstruction of the defect is based on the size.

1. *Obturator*: Most common and economical
2. Split skin grafting
3. *Soft tissue reconstruction*: Temporalis muscle flap/radial artery forearm flap
4. *Osseocutaneous flap reconstruction*: Fibula flap

TNM Staging

- *T1*: Restricted to any one anatomic subsite, with or without bony invasion
- *T2*: Invading two anatomic subsites in a single region or extending to involve an adjacent region within the nasoethmoidal complex, with or without invasion of bone
- *T3*: Invades the medial wall or floor of the orbital palate, maxillary sinus, or cribriform plate
- *T4a*: Invades any of the following: skin of nose or cheek, anterior orbital contents, minimal extension to anterior cranial fossa, pterygoid plates, sphenoid or frontal sinuses pterygoid plates
- *T4b*: Invades any of the following: orbital apex, middle cranial fossa, dura, brain, cranial nerves other than (V_2), nasopharynx, or clivus

Management Protocol NCCN Clinical Practice Guidelines In Oncology (NCCN Guidelines) for Ethmoid Tumors[3]

Depending on the evidence, the NCCN consensus for these recommendations may vary.

1. *Newly diagnosed T1–T2*: Surgical resection (preferred) **or** definitive radiation
2. *Newly diagnosed T3–T4a*: Surgical resection (preferred) **or** chemoradiation
3. *Newly diagnosed T4b or patient declines surgery*: Treatment depends on patient factors but may include chemoradiation **or** radiation **or** clinical trial

4. *Diagnosed after incomplete resection and gross residual disease*: Surgery (preferred) **or** radiation **or** chemoradiation

5. *Diagnosed after incomplete resection and no residual disease on physical exam, imaging, and/or endoscopy*: Radiation **or** surgery (if feasible)

Regional lymph nodes (N)

- *NX*: Cannot be assessed
- *N0*: No regional lymph node metastasis
- *N1*: Single ipsilateral lymph node is 3 cm or less in diameter
- *N2*: Single ipsilateral lymph node is >3 cm but <6 cm in diameter, or in multiple ipsilateral lymph node is <6 cm in greatest diameter, or in bilateral or contralateral lymph node is <6 cm in greatest diameter
- *N2a*: Single ipsilateral lymph node is >3 cm but <6 cm in diameter
- *N2b*: Multiple ipsilateral lymph node is <6 cm in diameter
- *N2c*: Bilateral or contralateral lymph node is <6 cm in diameter
- *N3*: Metastasis in a lymph node is >6 cm in diameter

Distant metastasis (M)

- *MX*: Metastasis cannot be assessed
- *M0*: No distant metastasis
- *M1*: Distant metastasis

TNM staging

- *Stage 0*: Tis N0 M0
- *Stage I*: T1 N0 M0
- *Stage II*: T2 N0 M0
- *Stage III*: T3 N0 M0
  - T1 N1 M0
  - T2 N1 M0
  - T3 N1 M0
- *Stage IVA*: T4a N0 M0
  - T4a N1 M0
  - T1 N2 M0
  - T2 N2 M0
  - T3 N2 M0
  - T4a N2 M0
- *Stage IVB*: T4b any N M0
  - Any T N3 M0
- *Stage IVC*: Any T, any N M1

REFERENCES

1. Watkinson J, Gilbert R. *Stell & Maran's textbook of head and neck surgery and oncology.* CRC Press; 2011 Dec 30.
2. McGregor IA, McGregor FM. *Cancer of the face and mouth: pathology and management for surgeons.* Churchill Livingstone; 1986.

3. Referenced with permission from the NCCN Guidelines® for Head and Neck Cancers V.2.2019 © National Comprehensive Cancer Network, Inc. 2019. All rights reserved. Accessed [July 12, 2019]. *Available online at* http://www.NCCN.org. NCCN makes no warranties of any kind whatsoever regarding their content, use or application and disclaims any responsibility for their application or use in any way.

15

Salivary Glands

Major Salivary Glands

Primary site
- *Tumors arising from major salivary glands*: They are staged according to the site of anatomic origin (Fig 15.1)

Regional lymph nodes
- Spread less common
- *Low-grade tumors*: They rarely metastasize to regional lymph nodes
- *Regional dissemination*: Intraglandular to adjacent lymph nodes then upper and mid-jugular nodes

Clinical staging
- *Assessment*: Soft tissues study from skull base to hyoid bone
- *Ca of submandibular and sublingual*: Cross-sectional imaging
- *MRI or CT scan*: To check the extent and bony invasion of the tumor

TNM classification

Primary tumor (T)
- *TX*: Cannot be assessed
- *T0*: No evidence of primary tumor
- *T1*: 2 cm or less in dimension with no extraparenchymal extension
- *T2*: >2 cm but <4 cm in dimension with no extraparenchymal extension
- *T3*: >4 cm and/or tumor with extraparenchymal extension
- *T4a*: Invades skin, mandible, ear canal, and/or facial nerve
- *T4b*: Invades skull base and/or pterygoid plates and/or encases carotid artery

Regional lymph nodes (N)
- *NX*: Cannot be assessed
- *N0*: No regional lymph node metastasis
- *N1*: Single ipsilateral lymph node, 3 cm or less in dimension
- *N2*: Single ipsilateral lymph node, >3 cm but <6 cm in dimension, or in multiple ipsilateral lymph nodes, <6 cm in dimension, or in bilateral or contralateral lymph nodes, <6 cm in dimension
- *N2a*: Single ipsilateral lymph node >3 cm but <6 cm in dimension
- *N2b*: Multiple ipsilateral lymph nodes, <6 cm in dimension
- *N2c*: Bilateral or contralateral lymph nodes, <6 cm in dimension
- *N3*: Metastasis in a lymph nodes, >6 cm in greatest dimension

Distant metastasis (M)
- *MX*: Metastasis cannot be assessed

DOI: 10.1201/9780367822019-15

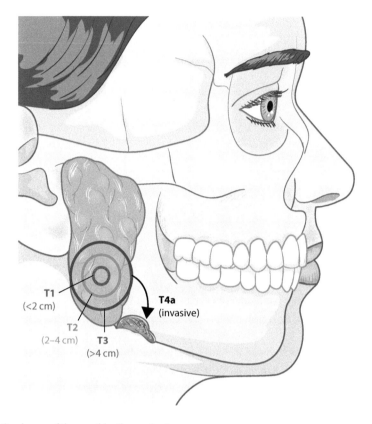

FIGURE 15.1 Carcinoma of the parotid salivary gland.

- *M0*: No distant metastasis
- *M1*: Distant metastasis

TNM staging

- *Stage 0*: Tis N0 M0
- *Stage I*: T1 N0 M0
- *Stage II*: T2 N0 M0
- *Stage III*: T3 N0 M0
  - T1 N1 M0
  - T2 N1 M0
  - T3 N1 M0
- *Stage IVA*: T4a N0 M0
  - T4a N1 M0
  - T1 N2 M0
  - T2 N2 M0
  - T3 N2 M0
  - T4a N2 M0
- *Stage IVB*: T4b any N M0
  - Any T N3 M0
- *Stage IVC*: Any T, any N M1

Management Protocol NCCN Clinical Practice Guidelines in Oncology (NCCN Guidelines) for Head and Neck Cancers V.2.2019 for Salivary Gland Tumors[1]

Depending on the evidence, NCCN consensus for these recommendations may vary.

1. *Clinically benign or carcinoma T1–T2*: Complete surgical resection
   a. If it's benign, follow up the patient.
   b. If it's of low grade and if there is tumor spillage/perineural invasion, consider adjuvant radiation.
   c. If it's adenoid cystic or intermediate- or high grade, give adjuvant radiation.
2. T3, T4a
   a. Check whether from parotid glands or other glands.
3. If parotid gland tumor
   a. *Clinical N0*: Parotidectomy with complete resection of tumor with/without neck dissection for high-grade tumors.
   b. *Clinical N+*: Parotidectomy with neck dissection.
4. Other salivary glands
   a. *Clinical N0*: Complete resection of tumor.
   b. *Clinical N+*: Complete resection of tumor and lymph node dissection.
      • After a resection of the tumor, if there is adenoid cystic carcinoma, give adjuvant radiation.
      • After a resection of the tumor, if there are positive margins/high-grade tumor/perineural invasion/lymph node metastasis/vascular invasion, give adjuvant radiation (preferred) **or** chemoradiation.
      • If there is incomplete resection, perform surgical re-resection (preferable) **or** definitive radiation **or** chemoradiation.

REFERENCE

1. Referenced with permission from the NCCN Guidelines for Head and Neck Cancers V.2.2019 © National Comprehensive Cancer Network, Inc. 2019. All rights reserved. Accessed [July 12, 2019]. *Available online at*: http://www.NCCN.org. NCCN makes no warranties of any kind whatsoever regarding their content, use or application and disclaims any responsibility for their application or use in any way.

16

Thyroid Gland

Thyroid

Primary site

- Thyroid gland

Stages of Cancer of the Thyroid

Once cancer of the thyroid cancer is diagnosed, there are various diagnostic tests done to confirm if there is distant metastasis. This is called staging. A surgeon needs to have an idea of the stage of the disease to plan the treatment (Figure 16.1)[1].

The stages for papillary cancers of the thyroid are as follows

Papillary and Follicular Thyroid Cancers in Patients Less Than 55 Years of Age

Stage I: Papillary and Follicular

- In stage I cancer of papillary and follicular type, the tumor is of any size that may be in the thyroid gland or may have spread to nearby tissues and lymph nodes. There is no distant metastasis.

Stage II: Papillary and Follicular

- In stage II cancer of papillary and follicular type, the tumor is of any size, and there is metastasis from thyroid gland to rest of the body, which includes lungs or bone, and may have spread to lymph nodes.

Papillary and Follicular Thyroid Cancer in Patients More Than 55 Years of Age

Stage I: Papillary and Follicular

- In stage I cancer of papillary and follicular type, tumor is found only in the thyroid and is smaller than or equal to 2 cm.

Stage II: Papillary and Follicular

- In stage II cancer of papillary and follicular type, tumor is only inside the thyroid gland, which is more than 2 cm but not more than 4 cm.

Stage III: Papillary and Follicular

In stage III cancers of papillary and follicular type, either of the following is seen:

- The tumor is more than 4 cm and only found inside the thyroid gland, or it is of any size and has spread to extra-thyroidal tissues just outside the thyroid, but not to cervical lymph nodes; or
- The tumor is of any size and may have spread to extra-thyroidal tissues just outside the thyroid gland and has spread to lymph nodes near the trachea or the larynx.

DOI: 10.1201/9780367822019-16

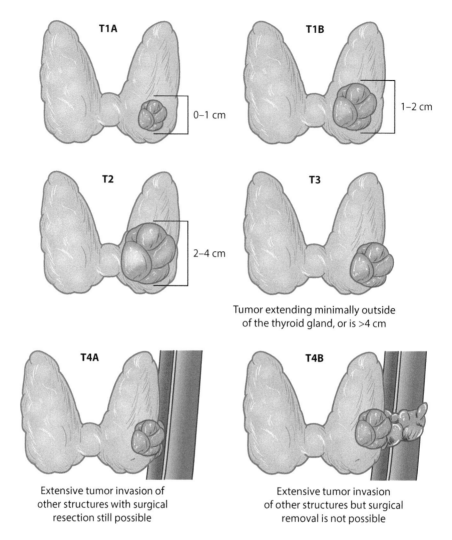

FIGURE 16.1 Carcinoma of the thyroid gland.

Stage IV: Papillary and Follicular
Stage IV cancers of papillary and follicular types are further divided into stages IVA, IVB, and IVC.

In *stage IVA*, either any of the following is seen:
- The tumor is of any size and has spread to extra-thyroidal tissues beneath the skin, the esophagus, the trachea, the larynx, and/or involving the recurrent laryngeal nerve. Tumor may have spread to adjacent cervical lymph nodes; or
- The tumor is of any size and may have spread to extra-thyroidal tissue. Metastasis on one or both sides of the neck lymph nodes or between the lungs is observed.
- In *stage IVB*, the tumor has spread to the tissue in front of the spinal column or has encircled the carotid artery or other blood vessels in the area between the lungs; metastasis to adjacent lymph nodes is present.
- In *stage IVC*, the tumor is of any size and has distant spread, such as the bones and lung and may have spread to lymph nodes.

Medullary Thyroid Cancer

Stage 0: Medullary thyroid cancer is diagnosed only with the help of a special screening test. No tumor can be found in the thyroid gland.

Stage I: Medullary thyroid cancer is diagnosed only in the thyroid gland and is 2 cm or less in diameter.

Stage II: In medullary thyroid cancer, either of the following is found:

- The tumor is more than 2 cm and present only in the thyroid gland; or
- The tumor is of any size and has spread to extra-thyroidal tissues, but not to the adjacent lymph nodes.

Stage III: In stage III medullary thyroid cancer, the tumor is of any size which has spread to lymph nodes near the larynx and the trachea and may have spread to extra-thyroidal tissues.

Stage IV: In stage IV cancers of papillary and follicular types is further divided into stages IVA, IVB, and IVC.

- In *stage IVA*, either any of the following is seen:
- The tumor is of any size and has spread to extra-thyroidal tissues beneath the skin, the esophagus, the trachea, the larynx, and/or involving the recurrent laryngeal nerve. Tumor may have spread to adjacent cervical lymph nodes; or
- The tumor is of any size and may have spread to extra-thyroidal tissue. Metastasis on one or both sides of the neck lymph nodes or between the lungs is seen.
- In *stage IVB*, the tumor has spread to the tissue in front of the spinal column or has encircled the carotid artery or other blood vessels in the area between the lungs; metastasis to adjacent lymph nodes is present.
- In *stage IVC*, the tumor is of any size and has distant spread, such as the bones and lung and may have spread to lymph nodes.

Anaplastic

Anaplastic thyroid cancers grow very quickly and spread usually within the neck when they are diagnosed or seen by the patient. Stage IV anaplastic thyroid cancer is divided into stages IVA, IVB, and IVC.

- In stage IVA, tumor is found in the thyroid and may have spread to adjacent lymph nodes.
- In stage IVB, tumor has spread to tissue just extra-thyroidal tissue and may have spread to adjacent lymph nodes.
- In stage IVC, tumor has spread to other parts of the body, such as the lungs and bones, and may have spread to lymph nodes.

Regional lymph nodes

- *First*: Paratracheal, laryngeal, and prelaryngeal (level VI)
- *Secondarily*: Mid and lower jugular, supraclavicular and upper deep jugular, and spinal accessory lymph nodes.
- *Upper mediastinal*: Occur frequently.
- Bilateral lymphatic spread is common.

Clinical staging

- *Assessment*: Indirect laryngoscopy to check vocal cord motion.
- *Imaging*: Radioisotope thyroid scans
  - Ultrasonography

- o   CT scan
- o   MRI scan
- •   *Diagnosis*: Needle or open biopsy.

Tumor, Node, Metastasis (TNM) classification

Primary tumor (T)
- •   *TX*: Tumor cannot be assessed
- •   *T0*: No evidence of primary tumor
- •   *T1*: Tumor ≤2 cm in dimension, limited to the thyroid
- •   *T2*: Tumor >2 cm but ≤4 cm in dimension, limited to the thyroid
- •   *T3*: Tumor >4 cm in dimension limited to the thyroid or any tumor with minimal extra-thyroid extension (e.g., extension to sternothyroid muscle or perithyroid soft tissues)
- •   *T4a*: Tumor of any size extending beyond the thyroid capsule to invade subcutaneous soft tissues, larynx, trachea, esophagus, or recurrent laryngeal nerve
- •   *T4b*: Tumor invades prevertebral fascia or encases carotid artery or mediastinal vessels
  - o   All anaplastic carcinomas are considered T4 tumors.
- •   *T4a*: Intrathyroidal anaplastic carcinoma are surgically resectable
- •   *T4b*: Extra-thyroidal anaplastic carcinoma are surgically unresectable

Regional lymph nodes (N)
Regional lymph nodes are in the central compartment, lateral cervical, and upper mediastinal lymph nodes.
- •   *NX*: Lymph nodes cannot be assessed
- •   *N0*: No regional lymph node metastasis
- •   *N1*: Regional lymph node metastasis
- •   *N1a*: Metastasis to level VI (paratracheal, pretracheal, and prelaryngeal/Delphian lymph nodes)
- •   *N1b*: Metastasis to unilateral or bilateral cervical or superior mediastinal lymph nodes
- •   *Distant metastasis (M)*:
- •   *MX*: Metastasis cannot be assessed.
- •   *M0*: No distant metastasis
- •   *M1*: Distant metastasis.

TNM staging
- •   Papillary or follicular thyroid cancer
  - •   Younger than 45 years
    - o   *Stage I*: Any T any N M0
    - o   *Stage II*: Any T any N M1
  - •   Age 45 years and older
    - o   *Stage I*: T1 N0 M0
    - o   *Stage II*: T2 N0 M0
    - o   *Stage III*: T3 N0 M0
      - –   T1 N1a M0
      - –   T2 N1a M0
      - –   T3 N1a M0
    - o   *Stage IVA*: T4a N0 M0
      - –   T4a N1a M0
      - –   T1 N1b M0

- – T2 N1b M0
- – T3 N1b M0
- – T4a N1b M0
  - ○ *Stage IVB*: T4b any N M0
  - ○ *Stage IVC*: Any T any N M1
- Anaplastic thyroid cancer
  - All anaplastic carcinomas are considered stage IV.
    - ○ *Stage IVA*: T4a, any N M0
    - ○ *Stage IVB*: T4b, any N M0
    - ○ *Stage IVC*: Any T, any N M1

Management

Surgical resection is the most common modality of treatment of cancer of the thyroid. A surgeon may remove the tumor using one of the following type of surgery:

- *Hemithyroidectomy*: It removes only the side of the thyroid gland where the tumor is located. Lymph nodes in the area may be biopsied to see if they contain tumor cells.
- *Near-total thyroidectomy*: It removes the entire thyroid gland except for a small part (misnomer).
- Total thyroidectomy removes the entire thyroid gland.
- Lymph node dissection removes lymph nodes in the neck that contain tumor.

Treatment by Stage

Treatment of cancer of the thyroid gland depends on the type and stage of the disease, patient's age, and overall health.

Standard/conventional treatment might be considered due to its effectiveness in patients, as published in past studies, or participation in any clinical trial may be considered. Not all the patients are cured with standard modality, and some of these standard treatments may have more side effects than are desired. For these particular reasons, clinical trials are designed to find better ways to manage these types of cancer patients which are based on the most up-to-date information. Clinical trials are ongoing in many parts of the country for some patients with cancer of the thyroid.

Stage I: Papillary Thyroid Cancer

Treatment may be any one of the following:

1. *Lobectomy*: Surgery to remove one lobe of the thyroid followed by hormone therapy. Radioactive iodine also may be given following surgery
2. *Total thyroidectomy*: Surgery to remove the thyroid

Stage I: Follicular Thyroid Cancer

Treatment may be one of the following:

1. *Total thyroidectomy*: Surgery to remove the thyroid
2. *Lobectomy*: Surgery to remove one lobe of the thyroid followed by hormone therapy. Radioactive iodine also may be given following surgery

Stage II: Papillary Thyroid Cancer

Treatment may be one of the following:

1. *Lobectomy*: Surgery to remove one lobe of the thyroid and lymph nodes that contain tumor, followed by hormone therapy. Radioactive iodine also may be given following surgery
2. *Total thyroidectomy*: Surgery to remove the thyroid

Stage II: Follicular Thyroid Cancer

Treatment may be one of the following:

1. *Total thyroidectomy*: Surgery to remove the thyroid
2. *Lobectomy*: Surgery to remove one lobe of the thyroid and lymph nodes that contain cancer, followed by hormone therapy. Radioactive iodine also may be given following surgery

Stage III: Papillary Thyroid Cancer

Treatment may be one of the following:

1. *Total thyroidectomy*: Surgery to remove the entire thyroid and lymph nodes where cancer has spread
2. Total thyroidectomy followed by radiation therapy with radioactive iodine or external beam radiation therapy (EBRT)

Stage III: Follicular Thyroid Cancer

Treatment may be one of the following:

1. *Total thyroidectomy*: Surgery to remove the entire thyroid and lymph nodes or other tissues around the thyroid where the cancer has spread
2. Total thyroidectomy followed by radioactive iodine or EBRT

Stage IV: Papillary Thyroid Cancer

Treatment may be one of the following:

1. Radioactive iodine
2. EBRT
3. Hormone therapy
4. A clinical trial of chemotherapy

Stage IV: Follicular Thyroid Cancer

Treatment may be one of the following:

1. Radioactive iodine
2. EBRT
3. Hormone therapy
4. A clinical trial of chemotherapy

Medullary Thyroid Cancer

Treatment is probably surgery to remove the entire thyroid gland; total thyroidectomy, unless there is distant metastasis. If lymph nodes in the neck contain cancer cells, the lymph nodes in the neck will be dissected (lymph node dissection). If there is distant metastasis, chemotherapy may be given.

Anaplastic Thyroid Cancer

Treatment may be one of the following:

1. Hemithyroidectomy removes the thyroid gland and the tissues surrounding it
2. Total thyroidectomy is done if the disease remains in the area of the thyroid
3. EBRT
4. Chemotherapy
5. Clinical trials studying new methods of treatment of thyroid cancer

Recurrent Thyroid Cancer

The choice of treatment modality depends on the type of thyroid gland cancer, previous treatment the patient had, and site of recurrence. Treatment may be one of the following:

1. Surgery with or without radioactive iodine
2. EBRT to relieve symptoms caused by the cancer
3. Chemotherapy
4. Radioactive iodine
5. Radiation therapy given during surgery
6. Clinical trials

REFERENCE

1. Watkinson J, Gilbert R. *Stell & Maran's textbook of head and neck surgery and oncology.* CRC Press; 2011 Dec 30.

17

Orbit and Eyelids

The TNM staging of different cancers of the orbit are as follows:

- Staging of *carcinoma of the lacrimal gland*
- Staging of *sarcoma of the orbit*
- Staging of *carcinoma of the eyelid*

Lacrimal Glands

Carcinoma of Lacrimal Glands

Lacrimal gland cancer is quite rare, which accounts for only about 2% of all orbital cancers (Figure 17.1)[1].

- Adenoid cystic carcinomas are the most common lacrimal gland cancers, accounting for about 30%–50% of all the cancers of lacrimal glands.

Other types of lacrimal malignant tumors of the lacrimal gland include the following:

- Carcinoma ex pleomorphic adenoma
  - A malignant pleomorphic adenoma can transform from a benign tumor that isn't completely resected by surgery.
- Adenocarcinoma
  - Lacrimal gland adenocarcinomas are very uncommon. They typically occur in people in their 50s.
- Mucoepidermoid carcinoma
  - Mucoepidermoid carcinomas tend to start in the ducts of the lacrimal gland. These tumors are rare.

TNM Staging

- *T1*: The tumor is of 2 cm or less in dimension whether or not it has extended into the orbital soft tissue outside the lacrimal gland.
- *T2*: The size of the tumor is between 2 and 4 cm in dimension.
- *T3*: The tumor is of >4 cm at its largest dimension.
- *T4*: The tumor invades into the layer of tissue covering the bone.
- *T4a*: The tumor invades into the periosteum of the orbit.
- *T4b*: The tumor invades into the bones of orbit.
- *T4c*: The tumor invades nearby structures such as the brain, sinus, temporal or pterygoid fossae.
- *Nx*: The regional lymph nodes cannot be evaluated.
- *N0*: There is no regional lymph node metastasis.
- *N1*: Regional lymph node metastasis present.
- *M0*: Distant metastasis cannot be assessed.

DOI: 10.1201/9780367822019-17

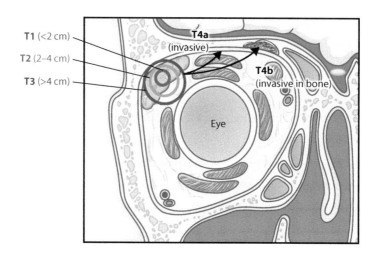

FIGURE 17.1   Carcinoma of the lacrimal glands (coronal section).

- *M1*: No distant metastasis.
- *M2*: Metastasis to other parts of the body.

Orbit

TNM Staging

- *T1*: The tumor is of 15 mm or less at its greatest dimension
- *T2*: The tumor is of more than 15 mm at its largest point but not invades the globe or bones surrounding the eye socket
- *T3*: The tumor can be of any size, which invades the orbital tissues and/or bones surrounding the eye socket
- *T4*: The tumor invades the globe or structures and the orbit (such as eyelids, temporal fossa, nasal cavity, sinuses, or the brain)
- *Nx*: The regional lymph nodes cannot be evaluated
- *N0*: There is no regional lymph node metastasis
- *N1*: Regional lymph node metastasis present
- *M0*: Distant metastasis cannot be assessed
- *M1*: No distant metastasis
- *M2*: Metastasis to other parts of the body

Sarcoma of the Orbit

Malignant orbital tumors may also occur as secondary cancers that have spread to the orbit from nearby adjacent structures, intraocular tumors of the eyeball, eyelids, sinuses or nasal cavity, and conjunctiva. The orbit is a small area. Tumors in the orbit can put pressure on the other structures within the eye, which can cause—bulging or protrusion of the eye (proptosis)—the most important signs of vision

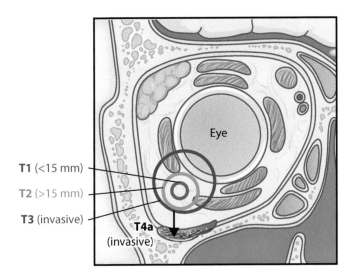

FIGURE 17.2   Sarcoma of the orbit (coronal section).

changes (such as double vision, blurred vision, or vision loss), and the abnormality of the pupil changes to eye muscle function pain (due to cancer in the orbital bone or nerves) (Figure17.2)[2,3].

Management

The treatment of primary orbital tumors often involves surgery. However, performing surgery for orbital tumors is difficult because of the limited space in the orbital area.

- Surgery on the orbit of the eye is called an orbitotomy. The surgical approach used depends on the size and location of the tumor.
- The surgeon will try to preserve the eye (ocular preservation) whenever possible.
- Enucleation or orbital exenteration may need to be done for more extensive tumors.
- External beam radiation therapy or chemotherapy may be an option after surgery, depending on the particular type of orbital tumors.

Eyelids

TNM Staging

- *T1*: The tumor is of <5-mm diameter length so cannot invade the margin of the eyelid or the tarsal plate
- *T2a*: These tumors invade the margin of the eyelid or the tarsal plate in the eyelid as their diameter lengths are between >5 mm and <10 mm
- *T3a*: The tumor is of > 20 mm at its largest diameter of the eyelid that invades nearby orbital or ocular structures
- *T3b*: Getting the tumor out would involve the removal of the eyeball
- *T4*: This type of tumors cannot be removed surgically because they get involved into the brain or extensive invasion of the skull/face, orbit, or ocular structures

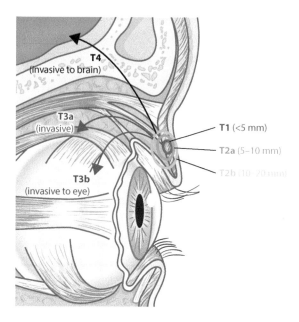

FIGURE 17.3   Carcinoma of eyelid (sagittal section).

Carcinoma of Eyelids

There are four main types of eyelid cancers (Figure 17.3)[4]:

Basal cell carcinoma (BCC)

- BCC is the very common type of tumors affecting the eyelid, contributing for about 85% of all the eyelid tumors. It is also the most common cancer type that occurs outside the orbit.
- BCC of the eyelid is usually observed affecting the adults but may also affect the younger people.
- These are the tumors that are related to the exposure of sun and are similar to BCC of the skin.
- Lower eyelid is the most common area for BCC.

Squamous cell carcinoma (SCC)

- SCC of the eyelid is very uncommon, accounting for about 5% of all tumors of eyelids.
- *Actinic keratoses or Bowen's disease:* Precancerous condition can cause SCC.
- They are also related to sun exposure and are similar to SCC of the skin.
- They behave more aggressively and are more likely to spread than BCC.

Sebaceous gland carcinoma (SGC)

- SGC occurs in the glands of the eyelid and accounts for up to 5% of all eyelid cancers and are very rare.
- It is more commonly found in women than in men and is seen most often in elderly population.
- These tumors grow most often on the upper eyelid then followed by the lower eyelid and in the caruncle.
- SGC can occur in the Meibomian glands, the glands of Zeis or the sebaceous glands of the caruncle.
- SGC is often diagnosed at an advanced stage because it can mimic benign conditions and can also grow aggressively.
- SGC may be multifocal (occurring in more than one anatomic site), so they always have a tendency to recur after the surgery.

Malignant melanoma

- Melanoma of the eyelid is a very rare tumor and is found in less than 1% of all cancers of eyelids.
- Melanoma of the eyelid behaves similar to that of the skin. So both the types of melanomas are staged and treated in the same way.

Management

The management for tumors of the eyelid usually involves surgical management.

- Surgical resection is done for the complete removal of the tumor along with a small amount of normal healthy tissues from around the tumor for oncologic clearance.
- Mohs surgery is a type of surgery used for the treatment of eyelid tumors in most situations.
- The Mohs surgery is a special kind of surgical method used to remove the tumor of eyelid layer by layer.
- These layers of tissue are then examined under a microscope until the excised tissue is found to be completely free of tumor cells.
- Only trained surgeons in the Mohs surgery can perform this type of surgery, so it may not be done at all treatment centers.
- Curettage and electrodessication can also be used to manage some small superficial BCC of the eyelid.
- Curettage and electrodesiccation is a surgical procedure that uses electric or a heat current to damage the cancerous tissue and thereby control bleeding.
- The destroyed tissue is then scraped off.
- If an eyelid tumor has invaded the eye orbit, orbital eccenteration might be necessary to perform.

If surgery leaves a defect of the eyelid, it can be repaired using reconstructive surgery.

Management options that may be used instead of surgery include the following:

- Cryosurgery that may be used for small tumors that are well defined.
- External beam radiation therapy may be used:
- as alternative to surgical management, if surgery would affect the person's facial esthetics;
- for recurrent or advanced tumors of eyelids that are difficult to remove or cannot be resected completely by surgery; and
- for people who are not well enough to have surgery or other treatments.
- Laser surgery is rarely used but may also be an option for some small tumors.
- Topical chemotherapy is rarely used but may be a choice of management in certain cases.

TNM Staging

- *Stage I*: Tis N0 M0
- *Stage IA*: T1 N0 M0
- *Stage IB*: T2a N0 M0
- *Stage IC*: T2b N0 M0
- *Stage II*: T3a N0 M0
- *Stage IIIA*: T3b N0 M0
- *Stage IIIB*: Any T N1 M0
- *Stage IIIC*: T4 Any N M0
- *Stage IV*: Any T Any N M1

REFERENCES

1. Woo KI, Yeom A, Esmaeli B. Management of lacrimal gland carcinoma: lessons from the literature in the past 40 years. *Ophthalmic Plastic and Reconstructive Surgery.* 2016 Jan 1;32(1):1–10.
2. Shields, J.A. and Baker Jr, H.L., 1989. Diagnosis and management of orbital tumors.
3. Shinder R, Al-Zubidi N, Esmaeli B. Survey of orbital tumors at a comprehensive cancer center in the United States. *Head & Neck.* 2011 May;33(5):610–4.
4. Cook Jr BE, Bartley GB. Treatment options and future prospects for the management of eyelid malignancies: an evidence-based update. *Ophthalmology.* 2001 Nov 1;108(11):2088–98.

18

Occult Primary

Definition

The occult primary is defined as a biopsy-proven cancer of the neck, which, even after a complete clinical and radiological workup that includes a proper physical examination, computed tomography (CT) scan, and triple endoscopy that combines esophagoscopy, laryngoscopy, and bronchoscopy, reveals or yields no primary demonstrable lesion in the head and neck region[1].

Epidemiology

The exact incidence of epidemiology is unknown, but the occult primary of the head and neck has an incidence of 3–7% presenting with squamous cell carcinoma of the neck.

The Risk of Lymph Node Metastasis Depends Upon

1. Density of lymphatic capillaries
2. Location of the primary tumor
3. Histological differentiation of the tumor
4. Size of the lesion
5. Recurrent or untreated lesions

Risk Groups for Occult Primary Based on the Location of Primary Tumor

- *Low risk*: <20% are T1 stage of cancers (ca.) of retromolar trigone (RMT), floor of mouth, gingiva, buccal mucosa, and hard palate.
- *Intermediate risk*: 20–30% are T1, T2 stages cancer of tongue, soft palate, floor of mouth, RMT, hard palate, and supraglottic larynx.
- *High risk*: >30% T1–T4 stages ca. of nasopharynx, pyriform sinus, and base of tongue.

Clinical Presentation

- Patients clinically present with a painless, solitary neck mass, most often noticed by the patient himself/herself.
- Masses are usually of at least 2–3 cm in size.
- Patients have usually gone through at least one course of oral antibiotics.
- Benign masses are also often solitary and painless.

Histological Differentiation

Most of the patients have either squamous cell carcinoma or poorly differentiated carcinoma.

- *Adenocarcinoma*: High chances of primary lesion might have arisen from below the clavicle.

DOI: 10.1201/9780367822019-18

Differential Diagnosis

Benign

- Developmental (i.e., thyroglossal duct cyst, branchial cleft cysts, or inclusion cysts)
- Inflammatory (i.e., lymphadenitis, benign reactive hyperplasia, and infected sebaceous cyst)
- Benign neoplasms (i.e., lipoma, fibroma, hemangioma, neurofibroma, parathyroid adenoma, or goiter)

Malignant

- Metastatic carcinoma, sarcoma, or melanoma
- Carotid body tumor
- Lymphoma, leukemia
- Primary major salivary gland tumor
- Thyroid cancer
- Parathyroid cancer
- Carcinoid
- Histiocytosis

Diagnostic Workup (Figure 18.1)

History: Complete systematic history of the patient has to be taken.

Physical examination: Proper and careful palpation of the neck and oral screening for any lesions have to be done. Careful clinical examination of the neck and supraclavicular regions with special attention to skin has to be done. Soft, rubbery nodules suggest lymphoma and leukemia, while hard, fixed masses suggest carcinoma.

Mirror and fiberoptic examinations enable doctors to view the following areas: Nasopharynx, oropharynx, nasopharynx, and larynx.

Important note: Open biopsy must be avoided unless the patient is planned for definitive surgical management.

Histological examination: Fine-needle aspiration cytology (FNAC) is the most appropriate thing that can be performed to have a diagnosis. If it's not squamous cell carcinoma, rule out for lymphoma, thyroid neoplasm, or melanoma.

Radiological studies: Chest imaging/CT with contrast (CECT)/MRI with gadolinium. Positron emission tomography-CT (PET-CT) scan is suggested if other tests do not reveal a primary.

Laboratory studies: Complete blood cell count and blood chemistry profile.

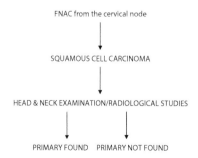

FLOWCHART 18.1 Workup for unknown primary.

If primary found, do the appropriate management; on the other hand, if it's not, take a PET-CT scan and proceed further.

Relationship of Nodal Location to Likely Disease

Nodes at certain levels more likely predict certain primaries.

Upper neck nodes are the most likely to be from head and neck cancers
- Subdigastric node may be virtually any head and neck primary, or a non-Hodgkin's lymphoma.
- Submandibular node suggests oral cavity, lip, nasal vestibule, or salivary gland primary.
- Submental nodes are uncommon and very rare.

Middle neck
- Likely primaries include larynx, hypopharynx, and less commonly esophagus, disease below clavicles or lymphoma.

Lower neck and supraclavicular nodes
- Most often metastatic from chest or abdomen, possibility of esophagus or lymphoma. A cervical node from primary head and neck cancer is uncommon at this level.

Parotid lymph nodes are more likely skin cancer than a primary parotid tumor.
Benign neck masses are most common except in supraclavicular lymph nodes.

Management

1. Treat as aggressive disease
2. Treat based on staging

Management Protocol NCCN Clinical Practice Guidelines in Oncology (NCCN Guidelines) for Head and Neck Cancers V.2.2019 for Occult Primary[2]

Depending on the evidence, NCCN consensus for these recommendations may vary:

1. *Node level I, II, III, upper V:*
   a. Examination under anesthesia
   b. Palpation and inspection
   c. Biopsy areas of clinical concern and tonsillectomy with/without lingual tonsillectomy
   d. Direct laryngoscopy and nasopharynx survey
2. *Node level IV and lower V:*
   a. Examination under anesthesia, including direct laryngoscopy, esophagoscopy
   b. Chest/abdominal/pelvic CT
   If primary found, treat as appropriate.
   If adenocarcinoma of neck node, thyroglobulin negative, calcitonin negative: Levels I-III are involved, perform neck dissection with parotidectomy.
   If levels IV and V are involved, evaluate for infraclavicular primary or perform neck dissection.
   If poorly differentiated or nonkeratinized squamous cell or not otherwise specified (NOS) or anaplastic (not thyroid) of neck node, perform definitive workup and treatment.
3. *Poorly differentiated or nonkeratinized squamous cell or not otherwise specified (NOS) or anaplastic (not thyroid) of neck node:*
   a. *Surgery with neck dissection:* Preferred for N1 disease **(or)**
   b. Radiation for <N2 disease **(or)**

c. Chemotherapy/radiation for N2 or N3 disease **(or)**

d. Induction chemotherapy followed by chemoradiation or radiation for N2 and N3 diseases
After b or c or d, if there is complete response, follow up the patient. If there is residual tumor in the neck, perform neck dissection.

4. *Post neck dissection:*

a. *N1 without extracapsular spread*: Give radiation or observe the patient

b. *N2, N3 without extracapsular spread*: Radiation or consider chemoradiation

c. *Extracapsular spread*: Chemoradiation or radiation

REFERENCES

1. Watkinson J, Gilbert R. *Stell & Maran's textbook of head and neck surgery and oncology.* CRC Press; 2011 Dec 30.

2. Referenced with permission from the NCCN Guidelines for Head and Neck Cancers V.2.2019 © National Comprehensive Cancer Network, Inc. 2019. All rights reserved. Accessed [July 12, 2019]. *Available online at*: http://www.NCCN.org. NCCN makes no warranties of any kind whatsoever regarding their content, use or application and disclaims any responsibility for their application or use in any way.

19

Management of Carotid Blowout

Definition

Carotid blowout syndrome (CBS) occurs due to the rupture of the carotid artery or any of its branches. It is considered to be among one of the most devastating complications associated with the management of head and neck cancers.

Etiology

Carotid blowout occurs in patients with head and neck cancers/recurrent tumors and post-radiation-induced necrosis or pharyngocutaneous fistulas. The reported incidence is 40% for neurologic morbidity and 60% for mortality rates associated with this complication. Patients with CBS can have a wide variety of clinical presentations due to the rupture of carotid artery, leading to acute hemorrhage or exposure of the carotid artery. The reported incidence is 4.3% for carotid rupture after radical neck dissection (RND)[1].

Classification

CBS is classified into three types:

1. Threatened
2. Impending
3. Acute

Life-threatening CBS blowout is defined as a rupture or exposure of carotid artery because of wound dehiscence or if radiographic findings are consistent with neoplastic invasion of the carotid artery system and with nonhemorrhagic pseudoaneurysm. Rupture is almost inevitable if the exposed blood vessel is not adequately and promptly covered with healthy vascularized tissue like the muscle. Impending carotid artery blowout consists of short acute episodes of bleeding that can be resolved spontaneously with conventional surgical packing.

Complete rupture of the vessel is likely certain because the intermittent hemorrhage might originate from a ruptured carotid artery with a pseudoaneurysm. Acute CBS is defined as an acute, profuse hemorrhage that is neither self-limiting nor can it be controlled with surgical packing. A complete rupture of the vessel can occur, and the patient's condition will deteriorate rapidly if stabilization and immediate resuscitation are not accomplished before definite management (Flowchart 19.1)[2].

Pathophysiology

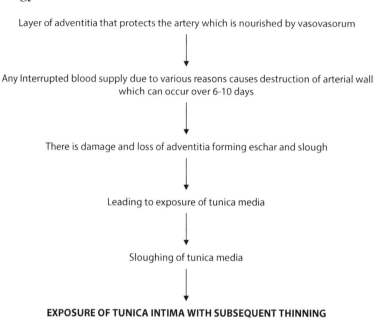

Layer of adventitia that protects the artery which is nourished by vasovasorum

↓

Any Interrupted blood supply due to various reasons causes destruction of arterial wall which can occur over 6-10 days

↓

There is damage and loss of adventitia forming eschar and slough

↓

Leading to exposure of tunica media

↓

Sloughing of tunica media

↓

EXPOSURE OF TUNICA INTIMA WITH SUBSEQUENT THINNING

FLOWCHART 19.1   Pathophysiology of carotid artery blowout.

Clinical Features

1. Herald bleeding or sentinel bleeding
   a. Minor bleeding from any site of the surgical wound, flap site, tracheostomy, or oral cavity.
   b. Process of erosion of blood vessel is gradual.
   c. This may be caused by a small rupture of the tunica intima at the site of the defect of the tunica which seals temporarily.
2. Pulsations from the artery or tracheostomy or flap site.
3. Ballooning of an artery.
4. Hemorrhage externally from the neck externally and internally within the oropharynx/directly into the airway or the site of tracheostomy.
5. Death due to:
   a. Hypovolemic shock is the most often the cause of death.
   b. Asphyxiation of blood may also be a contributory factor.
   c. Cerebral hypoxia.

Imaging Modalities

1. CT/MRI scan
2. Digital subtraction angiography (DSA)

   Selective catheterization of common carotid artery, external carotid artery, and/or internal carotid artery to detect active extravasation, pseudoaneurysm, and bleeding from tumor from the primary tumor or lymph node.

   Assess the intracranial circulation before intervention (surgery or endovascular)—selective carotid and vertebral injection and incomplete circle of Willis.

Management

1. Compression
2. Packing
3. Hemostatic material
4. Endovascular technique
5. Operative ligation

Surgical ligation of the common carotid artery or internal carotid artery is the conventional management for CBS. However, now, this approach is accompanied by unacceptably high rates of neurological complications and mortality. The high morbidity and mortality rates of this treatment are attributable to the following factors[2].

1. The surgical exploration of a field with area previously irradiated and surgery is technically difficult.
2. Without presurgical evaluation of the intracranial collateral circulation, surgical ligation of the carotid artery often results in thromboembolic events.
3. CBS often causes massive bleeding thereby leading to hypovolemia and the depletion of coagulation factors. Global cerebral ischemia and uncontrolled rebleeding can be encountered during the subsequent surgery and increasing the surgical risk.

Advantages

1. Often done in emergency setting hence less time for planning.
2. Ligate more proximally.
3. Ligation is preferable if there is multilevel rupture or multiple pseudoaneurysms.
4. Site of ligature must be always covered with a thick viable muscle flap which is not infected or diseased.
5. Preferable in clinically unstable patients.
6. Provides rapid securing of bleeding.
7. Technically less demanding compared to endovascular technique.

Ligation of common carotid artery

1. Carries significant neurologic morbidity and mortality due to intracranial cross circulation.
2. Ideally proceeded with balloon occlusion test or angiography of collateral circulation.
3. *Procedure*: Above the omohyoid
   a. Make a transverse incision on skin by palpating middle portion of sternocleidomastoid (SCM).
   b. Incise the fascia at anterior border of SCM longitudinally incised.
   c. Retract the SCM retracted posteriorly.
   d. Omohyoid tendon is retracted downwards.
   e. Carotid sheath exposed and dissected.
   f. Internal jugular vein is laterally retracted.
   g. Mobilize the common carotid artery (CCA), away from the vagus and ligate it.
4. *Procedure*: Below the omohyoid
   a. Make a transverse incision on skin by palpating the lower portion of SCM.
   b. Ligation of anterior jugular vein.
   c. Incise the fascia at anterior border of SCM longitudinally, omohyoid muscle is transected.
   d. Inferiorly, carotid sheath is covered by omoclavicular fascia which is exposed.

  e. Expose the carotid sheath and dissect it.

  f. Internal Jugular vein (IJV) is retracted laterally.

  g. Mobilize the CCA, away from the vagus and ligate CCA.

Muscle Flaps to Cover CCA

Levator scapulae flap is an option during RND. Care must be taken while dividing to prevent damage to the brachial plexus.

Endovascular management

1. Evolved since the 1980s.
2. Broadly classified into:
   a. *Deconstructive techniques*: It permanently occludes the vessel.
   b. *Reconstructive techniques*: It preserves the flow of the vessel.
3. Percutaneous balloon occlusion:
   a. Using a detachable balloon, it can be latex or silicone.
   b. Rapid occlusion of a large vessel can be achieved by this technique. This, it is more suitable for emergent conditions.
   c. Multiple balloons can be used in the same setting.
   d. 95% success rate in type 2 and 3 CBS.
4. Embolization with coil (platinum based), polyvinyl alcohol, or cyanoacrylate.

Reconstructive techniques[2]

1. Using overlapping or covered stents to diminish "porosity" between the stent struts.

   They promote sluggish flow and subsequent thrombosis around the stent. They allow blood to flow through stent and strengthen integrity of vessel. They are confirmed by second-look angiography.
2. Technically more demanding and time-consuming.
3. Indicated in patients at high risk for carotid occlusion.
   a. Angiographic documentation of incomplete circle of Willis
   b. Contralateral carotid artery occlusion.

Complications include rebleeding, thrombosis, and persistent infection.

REFERENCES

1. Cohen J, Rad I. Contemporary management of carotid blowout. *Current Opinion in Otolaryngology & Head and Neck Surgery*. 2004 Apr 1;12(2):110–5.
2. Chaloupka JC, Putman CM, Citardi MJ, Ross DA, Sasaki CT. Endovascular therapy for the carotid blowout syndrome in head and neck surgical patients: diagnostic and managerial considerations. *American Journal of Neuroradiology*. 1996 May 1;17(5):843–52.

20

Chemotherapy

Chemotherapy *kills cancer cells* or *modifies their growth*.

Classification of Chemotherapy Agents

- *Alkylating agents*: Cisplatin, nitrogen mustard, cyclophosphamide, chlorambucil, nitrosoureas
- *Antimetabolites*: Methotrexate, cytosine arabinoside, 5-fluorouracil, gemcitabine, hydroxyurea

Natural Products

- *Vinca alkaloids*: Vincristine, vinblastine, vinorelbine
- *Antibiotics*: Bleomycin, doxorubicin, mitomycin-c, dactinomycin
- *Taxanes*: Docetaxel, paclitaxel
- *Topoisomerase 1 inhibitors*: Irinotecan, topotecan
- *Hormones*: Tamoxifen, leuprolide

Chemotherapy Drugs Used in Head and Neck Cancer

- Cisplatin
- Carboplatin
- Methotrexate
- 5-Fluorouracil
- Paclitaxel
- Docetaxel
- Bleomycin

Principles of Chemotherapy[1]

- Determine that there is no better (more effective and safe) treatment available.
- The tumor must be susceptible to the drugs.
- The drugs and method of administration must not have intolerable local or systemic toxicity.
- Decide whether expected benefits (cure, palliation and the expected quality of life) justify the risk.
- Determine markers (symptoms, signs, laboratory measures) that will be observed to access the progress.
- With sensitive tumors, start the treatment early in the course of the disease to increase the likelihood of total cell kill.

DOI: 10.1201/9780367822019-20

- Cancer chemotherapy is more effective when tumor mass is small, than when the tumor cell burden is high.
- The drug must be present in sufficient concentration during the critical periods of the cells metabolic cycle.
- Chemotherapy is given in cycles to maximize tumor cell reduction.
- Repeat courses of high-dose chemotherapy with intervals for recovery of normal tissues.
- The administration of a combination of agents produces synergistic effects as well as an increase in the collective antitumor effect.
- Use adjuvant therapy to eliminate micrometastasis.
- The overall response rate to chemotherapy will depends on:
  - The type of agent(s) used
  - The number of agents used
  - The number of courses administered
  - Less histologically differentiated tumors may be more sensitive to chemotherapy
  - Previous surgery or radiotherapy may reduce the response to chemotherapy due to their adverse effects on blood supply
- Contraindications for use of chemotherapy:
  - Very advanced disease
  - Existing bone marrow depression
  - Presence of active infection

Types of Chemotherapy

- Combination chemotherapy
- Induction chemotherapy
- Concomitant chemoradiotherapy
- Adjuvant chemotherapy
- Sandwich chemotherapy
- Palliative chemotherapy
- Regional chemotherapy

Combination Therapy

The *combination of drugs is thought to be superior to single agents because resistance of cells to one agent may be sensitive to another.* In head and neck cancer, combinations have been based on *methotrexate* or *cisplatin*.

Induction Chemotherapy

The use of chemotherapy as the primary modality of management before definitive surgery or radio-therapy is referred to as *induction chemotherapy.*

Advantages

- Intact vascular bed allows for better drug delivery.
- Early eradication of regional and distant micrometastasis.
- Reduced tumor bulk facilitates surgery.

- Possibility of organ preservation.
- Chemosensitive tumors can be identified with a better prognosis and less extensive surgery, and radiation may be needed.
- Better performance status allows for better tolerance of chemotherapy.

Disadvantages

- Delay of potentially curative surgery
- Noncompliance after chemotherapy, missed opportunity for cure
- Over therapy, morbidity
- Increased cost
- Increased treatment duration

Concomitant Chemotherapy

In *concomitant chemoradiotherapy*, chemotherapy and radiation therapy are used simultaneously.

Rationale

- Radiation has an effect on sensitive cells in the irradiated field and thus is considered local therapy; chemotherapy acts locally and systemically outside the radiation field, which is referred as "spatial cooperation."
- Chemotherapy and radiation acts on different targets of tumor cells.
- Chemotherapy also acts against radioresistant hypoxic tumor cells.

Adjuvant Chemotherapy

Chemotherapy used in a patient rendered disease free by surgery and radiation therapy is called *adjuvant chemotherapy*. The aim of this is a reduction in recurrences. There is no evidence of the value of this approach in oral cancers at present.

Sandwich Chemotherapy

There is some evidence of reduced metastatic disease and nodal recurrence when chemotherapy is given after surgery and before radiotherapy.

Palliative Chemotherapy

This type of chemotherapy is used in patients deemed incurable. The main purpose is palliation.

Regional Chemotherapy

This is administered either as isolation perfusion or continuous intra-arterial infusion, both of which are designed to deliver large doses of anticancer drugs directly to the malignant tumors.

Mode of Action on Cell Cycle (Figure 20.1)

Chemotherapy and radiotherapy target actively dividing cells and the two most susceptible stages are the M-phase and S-phase of the cell cycle.

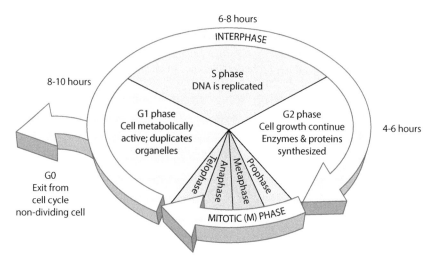

FIGURE 20.1   Mode of action of chemotherapy drugs on cell cycle.

Single-Agent Chemotherapy

- Methotrexate
- Cisplatin
- 5-Fluorouracil
- Bleomycin
- Vincristine
- Methotrexate is the most commonly used drug and can be administered by weekly IV injection at 40–60 mg/m^2

Chemotherapy Drugs in Head and Neck Cancer[2,3]

1. *Cisplatin*

   Cisplatin is a drug of an inorganic complex and is formed by a central atom of platinum, which is surrounded by chlorine and ammonia atoms in the "cis" position. It is an alkylating "agent which, after reacting with water," has a strong affinity for the negatively charged bases of RNA/DNA and causes cross-linking. There is a secondary effect in sensitizing cells to the effects of radiation.

   - IV infusion at 50–120 mg/m^2 body surface area is repeated at 3–5 weekly intervals.

2. *Methotrexate*

   Methotrexate is a dihydrofolate reductase inhibitor that prevents DNA and RNA synthesis. Folic acid may be used to "rescue" normal cells and enhance the therapeutic:toxic ratio. This is the most effective single agent and produces regression of disease in 50% of cases.

   - Intermittent IV administration is given in doses of 100 mg/m body surface area every 2–3 weeks. It can also be given intramuscularly (IM), orally or as a regional intra-arterial infusion into the superficial temporal or superior thyroid artery.

3. *5-Fluorouracil*

This is a pyrimidine antimetabolite specific for the S-phase of the cell cycle, which disrupts thymidine synthesis. It is found to have a 15% response rate in recurrent head and neck cancer. It can be given intravenously, orally, or as a continuous IV infusion.

- It is administered 1 g orally on alternate days (6 doses) then 1 g weekly or 12 mg/kg/day IV for 4 days.

4. *Paclitaxel*

Paclitaxel is one of the several cytoskeletal drugs that aim to target tubulin. There are defects in paclitaxel-treated cells that are present in mitotic spindle assembly, chromosome segregation, and also cell division. Unlike other chemotherapeutic agents that are tubulin-targeting drugs such as colchicine that inhibit microtubule assembly, paclitaxel stabilizes the microtubule polymer and protects it from disassembly. Chromosomes are thereby unable to achieve a metaphase spindle configuration, which in turn blocks the mitotic progression of mitosis and prolonged activation of the mitotic checkpoint triggered apoptosis or reversion to the G-phase of the cell cycle without cell division.

- Dosage of paclitaxel is 175 mg/m^2 IV.

Complications of Chemotherapy

- *Nausea/vomiting*: Antiemetics/Fluids
- *Diarrhea*: Antidiarrheals
- *Alopecia*: Turban/Prosthesis
- *Mucositis*: Mouth care, narcotics
- *Myelosuppression neutropenia*: Granulocyte colony-stimulating factor
- *Thrombocytopenia anemia*: Platelet transfusion
- *Nephrotoxicity*: Dialysis
- *Electrolyte wasting*: Repletion
- *Allergic reaction*: Antihistamines, steroids
- *Neurotoxicity*: Mainly supportive
- *Hepatotoxicity*: Mainly supportive

1. *Myelosuppression neutropenia (Flowchart 20.1):*
   - *Most serious and common toxicity*
   - *Limits the dose that can be employed*
2. *Causes*
   a. *Granulocytopenia, agranulocytosis (infection)*
   b. *Aplastic anemia*
   c. *Thrombocytopenia (bleeding tendencies)*

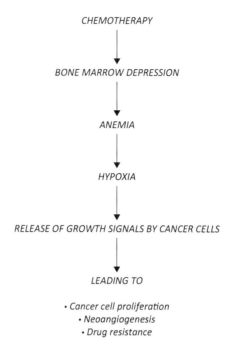

FLOWCHART 20.1   Myelosuppression neutropenia.

- Since cancerous cells thrive in a hypoxic environment, the hematocrit of cancer patient and their hemoglobin should be measured to maintain in the upper one-third of normal range before the commencement to the initiation of chemotherapy.

3. *Gastrointestinal tract*
   - Damage to gastrointestinal tract (GIT) mucosa and decrease in turnover rate causes nausea, stomatitis and vomiting.

4. *Skin*
   - Damage to the epithelium and decreased turnover rate leading to dermatitis.
   - Damage to cells in hair follicle leading to alopecia.

5. *Gonads and fetus*
   - Inhibition of gonadal cells and damage to fetus.

Important Notes

- *Standard chemotherapy consists of methotrexate, cisplatin or paclitaxel and is administered to patients with metastatic or recurrent head and neck cancer.*
- *Combination chemotherapy in recurrent disease may lead to improved response rates but without a major impact on survival.*
- *Induction chemotherapy for locally advanced head and neck cancer can produce high overall and complete response rates, but its impact on survival is minimal.*
- *Concomitant chemoradiotherapy for advanced head and neck cancer has a sound rationale. It is an appropriate treatment option for patients with unresectable disease.*
- *Because the outcome with standard therapy for many patients with advanced head and neck cancer is disappointing, participation in clinical trials should be strongly encouraged for all patients.*

REFERENCES

1. Schuller DE, Stem DW, Metch B, Mattox D, Mccracken JD. Preoperative chemotherapy in advanced resectable head and neck cancer: final report of the Southwest Oncology Group. *Laryngoscope*. 1988 Nov;98(11):1205–11.

2. Blanchard P, Bourhis J, Lacas B, Posner MR, Vermorken JB, Hernandez JJ, Bourredjem A, Calais G, Paccagnella A, Hitt R, Pignon JP. Taxane-cisplatin-fluorouracil as induction chemotherapy in locally advanced head and neck cancers: an individual patient data meta-analysis of the meta-analysis of chemotherapy in head and neck cancer group. *Journal of Clinical Oncology*. 2013 Aug 10;31(23):2854–60.

3. El-Sayed S, Nelson N. Adjuvant and adjunctive chemotherapy in the management of squamous cell carcinoma of the head and neck region: a meta-analysis of prospective and randomized trials. *Journal of Clinical Oncology*. 1996 Mar 1;14(3):838–47.

21

Radiotherapy

Definition

Radiotherapy, also called radiation therapy, and is one of the modalities used to manage diseases like cancer with ionizing radiation.

History

- November 8, 1895: William Conrad Roentgen discovered X-ray
- January 1896: Dr. Emile Grub—used radiotherapy for breast cancer
- 1898: Madam Curie discovered radium
- 1903 and 1906: Dr. Srabel and Dr. Abbe used radium into tumor mass for treatment of the cancer
- 1914: Sizilard: Used ionization chamber for output measurement
- 1920—Regaurd, Coutard, Baclesse: The use of fractionated radiation
- Rapid and major advances in radiotherapy techniques: Development of CO-60 machines linear accelerator, megavoltage therapy/super voltage therapy
- 1960s: CO-60, Cesium-136, Iridium-192, Palladium-103, Iodine-125 in brachytherapy were developed
- More recently: Use of hyperthermia, hyperbaric oxygen and neutron beam therapy were developed

Overview of Radiation

Radiotherapy uses high-energy photons or "quanta" of electromagnetic radiation to treat cancer. High-energy photons used in radiotherapy initially interact with tissue to produce high-energy electrons (500 keV to 10 MeV photon energies)-complex sequence of chemical reactions that generally involves free radicals within the cell cytoplasm[1,2].

"Direct" mechanisms and "indirect" mechanisms of action depend on the low- and high-energy radiation.

The most commonly used are X-rays, alpha and gamma rays. These radiations are concentrated onto the site of tumor to damage the DNA (critical target), but other elements like mitochondria also may be important.

Radiation doses are measured in terms of the deposited energy in a unit quantity of material which is specified as Gray, i.e., 1 joule being deposited per kg of material.

Principles of Treatment

- *Radical radiotherapy*
- *Palliative radiotherapy*
- *Multimodal treatment concept*

Principles of Radiotherapy

Radiotherapy is based on the basic premise that the fast-growing and metabolically hyperactive cancer cell is more sensitive to the high-energy radiation as compared with the normal cell.

The goal of radiotherapy is to sterilize the tumor and preserve adjacent normal tissue. Ionizing radiation deposits energy that injures or destroys cells by damaging their lethal dose for normal and abnormal tissues is about the same.

Normal tissues have a greater ability to repair sublethal damage between doses of radiation than the genetic material of neoplastic cells, making it impossible for these cells to continue to grow.

Sources of Radiation

In the mid-1970s, there was tremendous interest in the possible use of high-energy particles in radiotherapy. These particles include protons, neutrons, deuterons, stripped nuclei, and negative mesons.

- Gamma rays
- X-rays
    - Charged particles
- Protons
- Electrons
- *Negative*: Mesons
    - Uncharged particles
- Neutrons

Selection of Patients for Radiotherapy

- Physical condition of patient
- Probability of successfully completing treatment
- Site and histological type of tumor

The same type of tumor in a different location may have different biologic behavior and may respond differently to treatment. Histological type is an important predictor of radio-responsiveness.

Indications

- T1-T2-sized lesions
- T3, T4 locally advanced lesions

Postsurgical treatment

Only therapy if surgery not possible/contraindicated.

- Cervical lymph node
    - Elective treatment when there is no palpable lymph nodes present
    - Only treatment for clinically positive lymph nodes
    - Pre-surgical and postsurgical in combination with neck dissection for clinically N+ lymph nodes

Types of Radiotherapy

- *Brachytherapy*: This is the surgical placement of radioactive sources into/onto tumors.
- *Teletherapy (external beam radiotherapy)*: The source of radiation is at a distance from the body.

Orthovoltage Teletherapy

i. Primarily used to treat superficial lesions
ii. Orthovoltage machines produce low-energy X-rays that are absorbed near the skin surface.

It is difficult to treat deep-seated tumors without exceeding the tolerance dose of skin. Side effects are moist desquamation and skin necrosis.

Cobalt Teletherapy (Co)^{60}

i. Emits gamma rays; energy 10 times greater than orthovoltage
ii. Easier and safer to irradiate deep-seated tumors
iii. Maximum dose occurs 5 mm below skin surface; this "skin sparing" effect results in fewer skin reactions

Linear Accelerator External Beam Therapy (EBT)

i. Produces X-rays (photons) with energy 20 times greater than Cobalt-60
ii. Dose rate much greater; can treat more patients per day
iii. Depth of maximum dose varies from 5 mm to 1.5 cm. It has a tremendous skin-sparing effect
iv. EBT is replacing CO-60 radiotherapy for teletherapy

Systemic Radiotherapy/Internal Therapy

Treatment is done using a radio-pharmaceutical, which is internalized to produce the desired effect. These are radioisotopes, which are either injected or consumed as a drink.

Systemic radiation therapy is often used to treat thyroid cancers (I^{131}), adult non-Hodgkin's lymphomas, and polycythemia vera (P^{32}). Researchers are investigating agents to manage other types of cancer.

Ideal qualities of a radiopharmaceutical for RT are follows:

i. Effective half-life of the material must be in hours to days
ii. Medium/high energy (>1 meV)
iii. High target:nontarget ratio
iv. Minimal radiation dose to nuclear medicine personnel and the patient
v. Patient safety
vi. Readily available radiopharmaceutical

Preradiation Protocol

General

1. Avoid endodontic treatment procedure.
2. Extract teeth with periapical lesions, carious teeth.
3. Antibiotic use dependent on patient and treatment modality.
4. Fluoride (neutral sodium fluoride 1%) application on all teeth.

Weekly dental checkups during radiation therapy

- 14–21 days prior to radiation therapy, extractions must be done.
- Dental prophylaxis must be done.
- Restoration of large carious teeth.
- Any periodontal treatment must be avoided; extraction of teeth with more than 4–6-mm pockets, teeth of grade 2 mobility and furcation involvements of grade 2 or greater.
- Remove partially erupted third molars; don't remove full bony impacted teeth if surgical difficulty is more.

External Beam Radiotherapy

External beam radiotherapy is given as a series of short daily doses to head and neck cancer patients. Preparation time for radiotherapy often takes longer than the actual treatment itself for localizing the position of the tumor with the help of normal X-ray scans and computed tomography (CT) scans, which clearly give a three-dimensional picture of internal organs[3].

Steps

- *Mold and mold room*: Patient mold is prepared in a mold room.
- *Simulation*: Simulation includes marking of the particular area to be radiated, either temporarily or by tattooing, and all the procedures are done exactly in the same way with the patient positioned for the complete treatment. These values are transferred at the same time to the computer and fed into the treatment machine prior to start of treatment.
- *Planning*: The time taken in between the simulation and starting of the treatment is used for planning the treatment using the data collected in the simulator and CT scan, which is then transferred to the planning computer where appropriate calculations are done. This ensures the attainment and projection of the prescribed radiation dose to the cancer cells, while the dose to normal healthy tissue is kept to a minimum.
- *Treatment*: Blocks and shields are made of lead material to ensure that the radiation reaches only the specific target cancerous tissue. Port films are X-ray pictures taken on the treatment to ensure the precision of the target and so is three-dimensional computer software. Radiation shielding is mandatory for following organs: brain stem—above 54 Gy; mandible and TMJ—above 70 Gy; spinal cord—above 50 Gy; temporal lobe—above 60 Gy.
- The distance between the source and patient is 80–100 cm.
- *Dose*: The Radiation Therapy Oncology Group (RTOG) has conducted a dose-searching study to determine the maximum amount of dose that could be safely given for HNC patients. A amount of 1.2–2.0 Gy/day is advisable, and there must be at least a 6-hour interval between sequential radiation treatments to allow for repair of sublethal and potentially lethal damage in those tissues which have been radiated.

Extensive tissue damage as well as tumor recurrence can to be avoided.

1. Since the 1920s, fractionation has been the cornerstone of radiotherapy.
   The delivery of small multiple radiation doses in terms of fractionation always carries a lower risk of late complications than does the delivery of a single large dose.
   - Repair of tumor cells is hampered after sublethal damage to them.
   - Reoxygenation in tumor cells is 0.2%–100% according to type of tumor.
   - Possibility of synchronization of tumor cell population.

- Amelioration of adverse effects of tumor hypoxia.
- Normal tissue repair between fractions.

2. *Hypofractionation*
   - 6,500–7,000 cGy, 300–400 cGy 2–4 days/week
3. *Hyperfractionation*:
   - Multiple fraction 2–3 times a day 115–120 cGy/f up to 6,500–7,700 cGy
4. *Accelerated fractionation*
   - Accelerated fractionation is a modality of decreasing the overall time of management in an effort to reduce the repopulation of tumor cells in rapidly proliferating cancers.
5. *Concomitant-boost technique*
   - With this technique, treatment is delivered daily once for the first 3.5 weeks and then daily twice during the final 2–2.5 weeks, when tumor cells can begin to repopulate more quickly.

Advantages: Loco-regional control at 5 years was better with the twice-daily treatment (59% vs 40%) and better overall survival at 5 years with altered fractionation (40% vs 30%).

Brachytherapy

- Brachytherapy was introduced by Forstel in 1931 and was in use for many years. *Brachio* means *short*.
- *Types and Indications:*
- *Intracavitary*: Here the holder has the radioactive sources and inserted into the body organ like tongue.
- *Interstitial*: Here rods, wires or ribbons are directly inserted into the soft tissues of the body and are placed into the tumor bed, tongue, cheek, buccal mucosa.
- *Mold*: Skin tumors
- *High-dose rate brachytherapy: Sources used*—Cs^{137}, Ir^{192}, CO^{60}, 6,500 cGy 6 days in T1–T2 lesions
- *Dose*: About 3.0–3.5 Gy typically is given to a distance of around 1 cm from the periphery of the catheters every treatment, with two daily treatments are given about 6 hours apart. Each treatment time takes about 15–30 minutes.

Follow-Up Protocol[3,4]

2–4 weeks after completing radiotherapy:

- **1st year: 1–3 monthly**
- **2nd year: 2–4 monthly**
- **3rd and 4th years: 6 monthly**
- **At the end of 5th year: Discharge**

Treatment of Recurrence

- 90% of the tumor recurrences occur almost within the 2-year period.
- After 5 years, rate of recurrence is 8%. In such cases, debulking/radical surgery must be performed.
- Reirradiation of the recurrent tumors will be helpful only after one year. A 50–65Gy hyperfractionation or brachytherapy are used to improve the tissue tolerance to radiotherapy.

Posttreatment Protocol

- *Care of dentition*: Fluoride application and regular checkups.
- *Use of fluids*: To prevent kidney problems and pilocarpine 5 mg to compensate salivary dysfunction.
- Proper nutrition is required—high-protein food.
- Posttreatment follow-ups at regular and periodic intervals.
- Regular exercise.
- Counseling of the patient and group therapy and other modalities of treatment methods for proper emotional adaptation of the patient.
- Avoidance of all surgical procedures involving specially the bone for a minimum of 6 months.

Side Effects

- *Under 3,000 cGy*: Candidiasis, xerostomia, mucositis, and dysgeusia begin.
- *Over 3,000 cGy*: Xerostomia (mostly permanent) and taste dysgeusia, altered saliva (thick, more acidic, changed flora).
- *Over 5,000 cGy*: Trismus (reduced mouth opening). Major concerns for development of osteo-radionecrosis over a period of time.
- *Over 6,000–6,500 cGy* significant concerns for osteoradionecrosis.
- *Stimulated whole salivary flow rates*: A week after the beginning of RT, 57% decrease, and after 5 weeks (end of treatment) 76% decrease; years after, RT 95% decrease.
- Endocrine abnormalities like parathyroid adenoma, hypothyroidism, and hyperthyroidism.
- Atherosclerosis is mostly seen in doses more than 50 Gy.
- Progressive muscle fibrosis that may restrict the movements and function of the neck and shoulder. Sometimes trismus can also be seen.
- Visual impairment may occur due to cataract, radiation keratitis, cataract and optic neuritis.
- Secondary infection.
- Radiation-induced neuritis.
- Development of maxillofacial deformity and tooth developmental problems in children.

India has around 36 accelerator-based and 231 isotope-based radiation therapy machines. As per an evaluation by WHO, developing countries like India require one radiation therapy machine per million of population.

REFERENCES

1. Ang KK, Garden AS. *Radiotherapy for head and neck cancers: indications and techniques.* Lippincott Williams & Wilkins; 2006.
2. Rose-Ped AM, Bellm LA, Epstein JB, Trotti A, Gwede C, Fuchs HJ. Complications of radiation therapy for head and neck cancers: the patient's perspective. *Cancer Nursing.* 2002 Dec 1;25(6):461–7.
3. Bhide SA, Newbold KL, Harrington KJ, Nutting CM. Clinical evaluation of intensity-modulated radiotherapy for head and neck cancers. *British Journal of Radiology.* 2012 May;85(1013):487–94.
4. Horiot JC, Bontemps P, Van den Bogaert W, Le Fur R, van den Weijngaert D, Bolla M, Bernier J, Lusinchi A, Stuschke M, Lopez-Torrecilla J, Begg AC. Accelerated fractionation (AF) compared to conventional fractionation (CF) improves loco-regional control in the radiotherapy of advanced head and neck cancers: results of the EORTC 22851 randomized trial. *Radiotherapy and Oncology.* 1997 Aug 1;44(2):111–21.

22

Electrochemotherapy

Electrochemotherapy (ECT) is a specific type of chemotherapy that allows delivery and absorption of non-permeable drugs to the cell interior in recurrent or progressive cutaneous and subcutaneous tumors where salvage surgery becomes a challenge for the surgeon. It depends on the local application of intense and short electric pulses that transiently permeabilize the cell membrane, thus permitting the transport of chemotherapy molecules that are generally not permitted by the membrane.

Machine

Permeos ECT is a tumor treatment option used for treating cutaneous and subcutaneous tumors with any histology. Permeos is designed with respect to Indian conditions and has local technical support. It is recommended in neoadjuvant, adjuvant, and palliative treatment of tumors and for the management of difficult tumors. It can often deliver tumor healing even when other treatment modalities fail (Figure 22.1).

- Easy operation via touch screen
- Very simple menu logic
- Patient data and therapy parameters are stored
- Therapy progress is visualized via an integrated control channel just seconds before and after the pulses
- Electroporation is applied via eight pulses of 100 μs duration each
- Voltage is 1000 V

Mechanism of Permeos ECT

The Permeos tumor therapy electrodes are placed minimally invasively under the skin inside or around the tumor. Each session takes about 20 minutes and is commonly performed under either local anesthesia or general anesthesia depending on the scope of the application.

Steps:

1. A cytotoxic drug is injected all around the tumor cell.
2. The electrodes of Permeos tumor therapy are inserted inside or around the tumor. Short electric pulses are then delivered to the cell.
3. Prior calculated voltage electric pulses for duration open up small pores in the cell wall through which the active substance can penetrate into the cell. When the pulses stop, the pores get closed again.
4. When the pores are closed, the cytotoxic agent can unfold its effect with increased intensity within the tumor cell and destroy it.

The application of Permeos tumor therapy pulses amplifies the effect of the active substance, destroying the DNA strands and thus killing the tumor cell. The application also inhibits the tumor cell's blood supply. The shortage adds to the effect of the substance, further weakening the cell and accelerating its dieback.

DOI: 10.1201/9780367822019-22

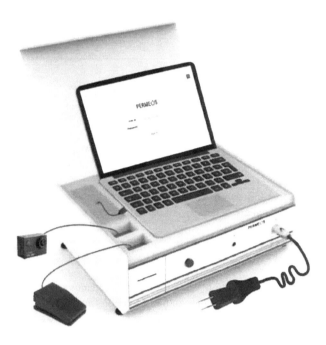

FIGURE 22.1 Electrochemotherapy machine.

Technique

The treatment is done by the injection of cisplatin intratumorally using a sterile needle. The dosage of cisplatin is approximately 1 mg/cm^3 of the size of tumor. In the case of large tumor nodules, cisplatin is injected in several different tumor areas in order to obtain complete and better distribution and absorption of the drug. Electric pulses are applied with Permeos-made needle electrodes. The distance between the electrodes is 6 mm. Electric pulse generator Permeos is used, which delivers electric pulses, amplitude/distance ratio 1100 V/cm, 10 mm long, with a frequency of 1 Hz (Figure 22.2).

Electric pulses are delivered in two sets of four pulses, which are in perpendicular direction with one second pause in between each set. Nodules that are larger than the distance between the electrodes are treated by consecutive multiple application of electric pulses to cover the whole tumor nodules. Immediate effects of the treatment are marks of the electrodes on the skin that disappeared after few minutes, unpleasant sensations that are predominantly caused by muscular contractions. The pain is bearable and hence patients do not really require pain control measures. The patients are then regularly assessed for their response to treatment in 2- to 4- week intervals. Some tumors need numerous treatments. Big tumors require another cycle every 4 weeks to remove the whole tumor mass. There is a varied observation time of patients depending on the inclusion time into the study ranging from a few weeks to up to one year[1].

Studies

Based on the multicenter ESOPE (European Standard Operation Procedures for Electrochemotherapy) in 2006, the ESOPE guidelines provide a systematic algorithm for the management of multiple metastatic cutaneous and subcutaneous nodules. In the ESOPE study, standard operating procedures for management were used and the results showed a complete response rate (CRR) of 73.7% in 171 cutaneous and subcutaneous, nodules metastases of different histopathology in 41 patients after a 5-month median follow-up period.

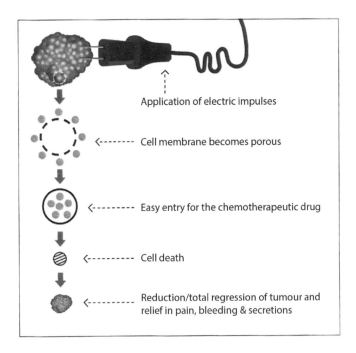

Application of electric impulses

<------- Cell membrane becomes porous

<-------- Easy entry for the chemotherapeutic drug

<--------- Cell death

<--------- Reduction/total regression of tumour and relief in pain, bleeding & secretions

FIGURE 22.2 Technique of Permeos.

Freidik Landstorm et al. in 2015[2] in Sweden with 26 patients, did long-term follow-up of patients who underwent ECT with intratumoral bleomycin in T1 and T2 head and neck cancers and nonmelanoma skin cancer. The primary objective of management is locoregional control and treatment safety. The secondary objective was survival and functional assessment. A possible selective effect in vitro of ECT on survival in different human cell types, normal and malignant, was also investigated. The local control rate in the 19 HNC patients managed with curative intent was 100% in a follow-up period of 60 months. Six patients had a complete response by ECT as a mono-modality treatment and the other six patients by ECT as well as adjuvant radiation therapy.

Out of seven patients, three patients expired from progressive disease and four patients expired from local recurrence, thus making the tumor-specific survival for 75%. The functional and safety outcome was very good in 15 patients who were treated with cancers of oral tongue but very poor in the patients who had tumors in the floor of mouth, buccal mucosa and base of tongue. Four patients of these six patients with nonmelanoma skin cancer had a complete response in 24 months after ECT management alone. The management in three patients was also organ and function sparing. One patient had a tumor persistent and another patient had a tumor recurrence after 30 months of treatment. There was also evidence for cell-type selectivity of ECT with bleomycin on cell survival in vitro. The survival was significantly higher in fibroblasts compared to endothelial and squamous cell carcinoma cells. ECT is a good modality for curative treatment, which merits further investigation but a very good option for adjuvant modality.

A study done on 20 patients, which included T1-T4a tumors, had similar results with ours. In this study, on 20 head and neck carcinoma patients, ECT was used to treat tumor nodules with cisplatin injected intratumorally. Responses of the patients were evaluated based on the regression in the size (dimension) of the lesion. Out of these, 12 patients had clinical response of more than 60%, 5 patients had between 50 and 60%. Three patients had less than 50% clinical response; however, an overall clinical response rate in our study was 63.5% (Figures 22.3 and 22.4).

Positioning of multiple electrodes, and subsequent delivery of pulses, can be performed during a session to manage the lesion, provided that drug concentration is sufficient enough to electroporate it. Treatment can be repeated for weeks or months to achieve regression of large tumor lesions. Reduction

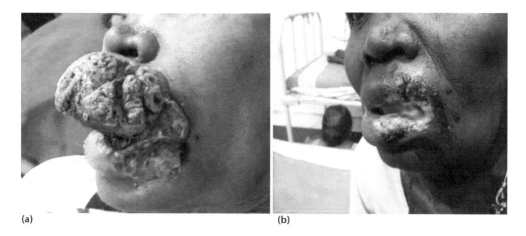

(a)   (b)

FIGURE 22.3   Fungating lesion of the lip: (a) Pre-ECT and (b) after 2 weekly sessions.

in the size of tumors has been achieved with ECT faster and much more efficiently than conventional chemotherapy. ECT is equally effective regardless of the tumor type and size of the nodules treated. Side effects of ECT are minor and acceptable.

Regarding the treatment procedure, ECT is very quick and easy to perform and not very expensive. The requirements are appropriate for the preparation of patient management with an electric pulse generator with sets of different electrodes that are used according to different sizes of tumor nodules. After the treatment, patients generally do not require any special attention or any kind of medications. Cisplatin was very successful to control the growth of the nodules treated. Tumors were regressed in most cases within 4 to 6 weeks, when superficial scab fell off. There was a slight depigmentation of the skin; however, it had a good cosmetic effect.

Apart from the advantages, there are also some disadvantages of ECT. For most patients, pain is a limiting factor. Pain can be avoided by applying the electric pulses after lifting the treated tumor nodule. In addition, it was observed that patients who were obese had less sensation due to less adipose tissue, which prevented the distribution of the electric field deeper into the underlying tissue; thereby muscle contractions were less. There was also a difference in sensations between the electrodes, which had a smaller gap of around 4 mm than those electrodes that had a bigger gap of 7 mm; hence, lower electric field intensity was required for electrodes with a smaller gap for tissue electroporation. ECT is a local treatment that can be very effective in the management of small tumor lesions that are not bigger than 30 cm

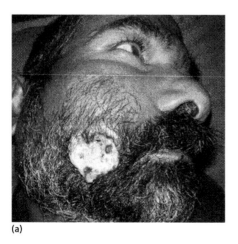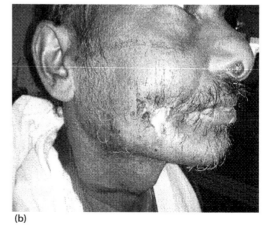

(a)   (b)

FIGURE 22.4   Fungating lesion of cheek: (a) Pre-ECT and (b) after one session.

in diameter. Therefore, it can be more effective in those patients who have very few or up to 15 lesions as skin metastases. In the case of more tumor nodules, ECT cannot be performed on all nodules in one session. ECT is, however, effective on those skin nodules that were treated but has no effect on the general progression of the disease. Due to occasional fast progression of the metastatic disease, new nodules emerge very soon, which were not seen in previous ECT sessions. ECT can be performed on these new nodules, and taken collectively, it can be effective in local control of the disease but does not affect the general progression of the disease[2].

Presently, the electrodes that are used are effective in the management of superficial nodules while they are not quite appropriate for nodules that are deeply located. Bigger nodules often require the use of several sessions of electric pulses and also various sessions of treatment in order to cover the whole area of tumor and to be able to remove deeper layers of the tumor. The use of ECT is doubtful when it is used to treat nodules/lesions that are larger than 30 cm in diameter and thicker than 5 cm.

ECT is one of the modalities of neoadjuvant/adjuvant treatment in locally recurrent/advanced disease patients. ECT is one of the modalities of treatment in locally recurrent disease patients when all the other options have been failed. It is not the only biomedical application of tissue electroporation, but also it has to be envisioned as the first step toward a wide use of electroporation in clinical application, predominantly in transdermal drug delivery and electrogene therapy[3].

REFERENCES

1. Mir LM, Orlowski S. Mechanisms of electrochemotherapy. *Advanced Drug Delivery Reviews.* 1999 Jan 4;35(1):107–18.
2. Heller R, Gilbert R, Jaroszeski MJ. Clinical applications of electrochemotherapy. *Advanced Drug Delivery Reviews.* 1999 Jan 4;35(1):119–29.
3. Bertino G, Sersa G, De Terlizzi F, Occhini A, Plaschke CC, Groselj A, Langdon C, Grau JJ, McCaul JA, Heuveling D, Cemazar M. European Research on Electrochemotherapy in Head and Neck Cancer (EURECA) project: results of the treatment of skin cancer. *European Journal of Cancer.* 2016 Aug 1; 63:41–52.

23

Targeted Therapy, Immunotherapy, and Gene Therapy

Targeted Therapy

In head and neck cancer (HNC), EGFR overexpression has been studied with a high locoregional recurrence rates and patients' poor survival. Although EGFR is overexpressed in more than 90% of HNC, only a limited group of these cancers demonstrate amplified copy numbers or mutational activation of the *EGFR* gene. Activation of EGFR in HNC is driven in part by its high expression of ligands, which helps in production of powerful paracrine and autocrine loops. Binding of these ligands to EGFR induces EGFR dimerization and autophosphorylation of its intracellular kinase domain, thereby leading to activation of multiple oncogenic pathways[1].

Targeted therapy is playing a key role at various areas along this signal transduction sequence in an effort to block EGFR function. Cetuximab which is a monoclonal antibody is directed against the extracellular receptor domain that seeks to block binding of these ligands and prevent dimerization of receptor, which induces receptor degradation and initiates the antitumoral response of immune system. Tyrosine kinase inhibitors such as gefitinib and erlotinib are small molecules but interact with the cellular domain of EGFR and cause inhibition of phosphorylation function. EGFR gene silencing can be done by numerous posttranscriptional strategies that include the use of sequence-specific antisense oligodeoxynucleotides and small interfering RNAs. Antisense oligodeoxynucleotides mainly consist of strands of antisense DNA that bind complementary EGFR mRNA and block the synthesis. Small interfering RNAs are short double-stranded RNAs that bind a specific mRNA, triggering its destruction via the RNA interference pathway.

Despite the importance of EGFR overexpression in head and neck tumorigenesis, EGFR blockade acting as monotherapy has been only partially successful in the management of patients with HNC. The limited use of monotherapy is not very surprising due to the divergency and complexity of signaling pathways that help in tumor growth, invasion, and tumor metastasis. Accordingly, there have been recent developments to combine EGFR blockade with other nontraditional and traditional management modalities, which includes the blockade of EGFR-independent signaling pathways.

Cetuximab, a drug of choice, is often used in combination with radiotherapy and has recently gained importance in improving locoregional control and survival of the patient with advanced HNC. Additional clinical trials conclude that cetuximab, along with other inhibitors of EGFR, may increase the effects of platinum-based chemotherapy. There are ongoing efforts that optimize blockade of EGFR by combining agents with specific but nonoverlapping anti-EGFR activity, such as the combination of tyrosine kinase inhibitors and anti-EGFR monoclonal antibodies. Another strategy that involves the concomitant targeting of signaling pathways is the blockade of EFGR-independent pathway, which may intersect the EGFR network pathway. EGFR resistance, at one side, has been attributed, in part, with increased levels of vascular endothelial growth factor (VEGF). This current finding, in turn, has initiated interest in the use of dual inhibitors of both the VEGF and EGFR receptors[2].

Immunotherapy

Immunocompromised patients are more likely to develop HNC, and tumors occurring in these patients tend to have a poor response. This can worsen the prognosis and has been documented in multiple clinical trials evaluating patients following hematopoietic stem-cell and solid organ transplantations. Once the patient develops HNCs, an endogenous host immune response is prognostic, as has been studied and identified for multiple tumor types. T-cell infiltration in both populations of CD8 and CD4 was identified to be prognostic in tongue-base and tonsillar SCCs. CD8 T cells as well as CD20 B cells were found in lymph nodes and prognostic in oropharyngeal and hypopharyngeal cancers. Interestingly, in his study, infiltration of these T cells into the primary tumor disease was not found to be prognostic.

CD8 T cells were found to be associated with metastases of lymph nodes, clinical stage, and tumor size in oral cavity cancers. Expression of ligands of immune checkpoint and their receptors has been further found to be significant and related with prognosis. One study documented that PD-1 infiltrates T cells in HPV-associated oropharyngeal cancer as a favorable prognostic factor. In recent studies of patients with oral cavity and oropharynx cancers, expression of PD-L1 was not found to be prognostic nor was indicative of any distant metastases but not related to local recurrence or overall survival of the patient. The clearance of oncogenic viruses is also related with outcome in malignancies which are virally induced. There are circulating EBV DNA that are found to be prognostic when quantified both pre- and post-definitive treatment, and also there are plans to use these titers of DNA after definitive chemoradiation to help the selected patients to recover for adjuvant chemotherapy following definitive chemoradiation in an upcoming cooperative group study. Similarly, another study of HPV-associated oropharyngeal cancer patients clearly demonstrated that the most of the patients who are successfully treated no longer harbor any evidence of oral infection post 1-year follow-up after the treatment[3].

There are clinical trials going on for plethora of immunotherapies for the management of established malignancies of the head and neck. These trials include pathways and approaches to vaccine production, adoptive T-cell therapy, and the use of certain targeted agents such as inhibition of immune checkpoints. A detailed explanation of this promising area is beyond the scope of this handbook, but some are described below.

Vaccines that target HPV are also being studied and explored for a wide variety of premalignant and malignant gynecologic diseases, and these conclusive findings could potentially be applied for HNC which are HPV-associated. Strategies for vaccination are also being studied and researched in HPV-negative malignancies. Preliminary testing of a dendritic cell vaccine that targets the p53 epitopes was recently published. The potential use of vaccination to prevent malignancies of the head and neck which are induced virally has been studied and described, however, vaccines that manage established disease are also under research. The bivalent and quadrivalent HPV vaccines targeting against proteins, which mediate viral entry into cells, are hence not expected to have efficacy to prevent HNC following initial infection. However, cancers mediated by HPV such as oropharyngeal cancer patients do express specific and typical targets such as the E6 and E7 oncogenic proteins which can be exploited by strategies of vaccination. Unlike many other potential vaccine targets include exogenous proteins; consequently, it can be easier to generate an antitumor immune response to overcome immune tolerance. Moreover, any immune reaction directed against these antigens would be expected to spare normal host tissue. Given their importance in oncogenes, these oncogenic proteins associated virally tend to be relatively conserved across individual cancers. This relative conservation in epitopes is against the more pleiotropic and variable mutations that are seen in oncogenes in nonvirally associated malignancy.

Immunotherapy, which is mediated by T cells, is also an attractive management strategy for virally induced cancers. Adoptive T-cell therapy directed against EBV antigens has met with minimal success for the management of EBV-mediated posttransplant lymphoproliferative disorders (PTLD). Unfortunately, EBV-associated nasopharyngeal cancers when compared with PTLD express lesser Epstein–Barr nuclear antigens (EBNA) and have lesser overall immunogenicity. Consequently, strategies which target-specific antigens are more often expressed such as LMP1-2 and EBNA1 may be the most efficacious. Current research studies have shown the feasibility of adoptive T-cell therapy that is directed against HPV-16 by demonstrating the ability of the transferred T cells to help to reactivate and expand specific E6/E7 T cells in more than 60% of oropharyngeal cancer patients who are tested.

Transfer of T cells with the help of engineered chimeric antigen receptors (CAR T cells) has been studied and tested in multiple types of tumors that could be used in the management of HNC. Although specific data for HNC are currently limited, EGFR can be engineered with T cells. EGFR expressed on HNC for about 90%, and the monoclonal antibody is cetuximab that targets EGFR, has clearly been demonstrated for overall survival benefit in malignancies of the head and neck. Although this is potentially effective, CAR T cells that have a great affinity toward EGFR could then have detrimental side effects given the widespread EGFR expression.

Immunotherapies activate an immune response that is dormant and often directed toward immune-activating ligands and checkpoint inhibitors. Toll-like receptor ligands could potentially enhance activation of immune system and have been tested in combination with cetuximab for malignancies of the head and neck, which has promising results in animal models. Inhibitors of the immune checkpoint receptors such as CTLA-4 and PD-1, as well as PD-L1 inhibitors, are being tested actively.

As described primarily, expression of PD-L1 has been identified on multiple subsites of head and neck tumors, and the expression of this PD-1 ligand can be predictive of a response to management that inhibits the PD-1 axis. Preliminary results of the study that included 60 patients with metastatic malignancy of the head and neck enrolled in the phase I study evaluating pembrolizumab, which is PD-1 inhibitor in various types of malignancy, were recently presented. This study required patients to have tumors which demonstrated expression of PD-L1. With limited follow-up of the study, there were no serious adverse events related to the drug, and responses were recorded in patients with both non-HPV-associated and HPV-related tumors. Decreased tumor burden was reported in 51% of patients with a 20% response rate. Interestingly, patients who had tumors that demonstrated the expression of PD-L1 were also the patients more likely to respond to treatment (46% response rate as compared with 11%).

Gene Therapy

For a normal cell to become "cancerous" or gain malignant potential, it has to undergo certain epigenetic changes or mutations. They are somatic changes, mostly brought by a specific incidence or environmental factors, with only a minimal proportion being caused by inherited factors. The normal cycle of cell is regulated by various genetic segments that include proto-oncogenes and tumor suppressor genes held in state of equilibrium. Any kind of upset to this equilibrium by increased expression of (proto-) oncogene or any reduction in expression of tumor suppressor gene leads to aberrant proliferation and, hence, causes "cancer". On a cellular level, the prominent changes of a cancerous cell are as follows: Self-sufficiency can be seen in signals of growth, anti-growth signals insensitivity, sustained angiogenesis, limitless replicative potential, evading apoptosis, tissue invasion and metastases. Gene therapy of cancer is based on the gene insertion called transfection into a cell. This formed new DNA is then "transcribed" to make mRNA which has encoded to a specific type of protein that is made from the process of translation[4].

As the whole mapping of the human genome has been done and can select from a varied number of genes available. This kind of gene therapy can be identified as "corrective", "immunomodulatory", or "cytoreductive". A cancer gene is a gene that is causally implicated in oncogenesis. It can be either a tumor suppressor gene or an oncogene. To date, there are 291 reported oncogenes. According to English literature, more than 1% of all the genes are in the human genome while 90% of cancer genes show somatic mutations in cancer and 20% show germline mutations while 10% show both of the mutations.

Corrective gene therapy acts by either blocking the oncogenes or by replacing tumor suppressor genes. In the case of tumor suppressor genes, the main motto is to express a gene under the control of a suitable promoter, which can enhance the production of specific therapeutic product of genes. The typical type of tumor suppressor gene in HNSCC and most other types of cancer is p53, which has built a mechanism of safety involving every cell. If the genetic material within the cell is damaged, the material may cause it to behave in a very abnormal way, as p53 gene stops the cell cycle by binding to DNA. If the damage is unrepairable, it triggers apoptosis of the cell. P53 gene alteration results in continued multiplication and propagation of the damaged cell line. P53 gene replacement results in increased radiochemosensitivity and reduced HNSCC growth.

An US trial in recurrent advanced HNSCC showed a 50% positive response in most of the cases. China has a commercially available gene therapy agent based on p53 for HNSCC. This is in the form of Gendicine manufactured from a Shenzhen SiBiono GeneTech. Phase I trials were carried, which included 12 patients with advanced laryngeal cancers; there was a claimed response, without any 5-year relapse rate in 11 of the 12 patients. In phase II and III clinical trials, radiotherapy and chemotherapy were shown to have synergistic effects. One hundred fifty-three HNSCC patients of which 77% of the patients were in stage III or IV were randomized to receive radiation primarily or in combination with Gendicine. Those patients who received isolated gene therapy in addition to radiation therapy had a 93% response rate with complete remission of the disease in 64% of patients as compared to 79% and 19%, respectively, in the radiotherapy group. To date it has been administered by various routes to more than 2500 cancer patients with a variety of cancers.

Cytoreductive gene therapy targets directly or indirectly to kill the cancerous cell rather than correcting the underlying genetic defect. Though there can be many genetic defects up until the time the cancer cells become apparent, this can be a logical approach. This can be done by adding the effects of other anticancer therapies such as chemotherapy, concentrating cytotoxic agents in cancerous cells that interfere with the tumor's blood supply or induce apoptosis.

The body's own immune system helps to clear HNSCC cells by introducing a gene into these cancerous cells, and does not affect the normal cells, that produces a foreign protein on the surface of cell. This synthesized tumor-specific antigen allows the cell to be visualized, identifies, and destroyed by the body's immune system. Cytokines or immune regulatory proteins can also be introduced into the HNSCC cells to stimulate and enhance the body's own immune response with regards to the tumor cells. Cytokine gene transfer can be performed in vivo where these cancer cells or immune cells are transferred into the body, or ex vivo where the cells are removed from the body for transfection and replaced back into the same body. There is a wide range of acceptance of immunotherapy in melanoma, lymphoma, and some virally induced malignancies.

Gene therapy can also be used as a vaccine against the antigens that are expressed by HNSCC cells. A specific type of antigen gene is injected into cancer cells, thereby guiding the host body to recognize them and then stimulate an immune response against the tumor cells. The major problem is the insufficiency of reliable antigens to the tumor specific type of tumor. Another approach to vaccination is to add an antigen gene that can produce a co-stimulatory molecule. This co-stimulatory molecule is essential for the tumor cell and produces an immune response inside the body.

Gene therapy in HNSCC remains limited to trials but seems likely to be widely accepted in clinical application in combination with present conventional modalities. Single-cell cancer type in a single individual is heterogeneous at the molecular level. The subtyping of these head and neck malignancies is still in its earlier stages. When more clinical studies are done, more specific gene therapies will be able to be tailored accordingly. Across the globe, there are over 1000 clinical trials of gene therapy to date which are in progress. More than 700 trials of these are for cancer, of which 54 trials are for HNSCC.

Administration of this vaccine is primarily done by viral vectors that are injected intra-tumorally. If the difficulties with systemic administration of vectors can overcome, the probability of treating metastatic head and neck disease would become a realistic proposition. Safety and efficacy of the genetic therapies is undoubtedly a primary concern and a rate-limiting factor to its widespread introduction. The first "successful" gene therapy agent was used in severe combined immunodeficiency (SCID) that resulted in at least two cancer patients later developing a leukemic type disorder. Trials are usually performed in cancer patients who are in preterminal stage to minimize the impact of adverse effects when balanced against the potential gain.

REFERENCES

1. Williams MD. Integration of biomarkers including molecular targeted therapies in head and neck cancer. *Head and Neck Pathology.* 2010 Mar 1;4(1):62–9.
2. Kundu SK, Nestor M. Targeted therapy in head and neck cancer. *Tumor Biology.* 2012 Jun 1;33(3):707–21.
3. Newbill ET, Johns ME. Immunology of head and neck cancers. *CRC Critical Reviews in Clinical Laboratory Sciences.* 1983 Jan 1;19(1):1–25.
4. Gleich LL. Gene therapy for head and neck cancer. *Laryngoscope.* 2000 May;110(5):708–26.

24

Robotic Surgery of Head and Neck Cancers

Anatomical Areas of Use

Transoral robotic surgery (TORS) may be used for both benign and malignant tumors of the palate, the base of the tongue, the palatine tonsils, the lateral and posterior pharyngeal wall, and from the tumors of parapharyngeal space, cancers of the larynx and hypopharynx. The main contraindications for TORS are trismus leading to incomplete visualization and accessibility of the lesion, involvement of bone, such as mandible, tumors involving more than 50% of the area of the base of the tongue or tumors of the posterior pharyngeal wall, tumors involving internal carotid artery or any involvement of prevertebral fascia.

Robotic System

The da Vinci TORS Surgical System is made of three major pieces of equipment:

A designed console for operating surgeon,
A robotic cart equipped of patient-side with four robotic arms, and
A very high-definition three-dimensional vision cart.

Articulating surgical instruments are then mounted on the arms of the robot, which are later introduced through the oral cavity inside the patient's upper aerodigestive tract and controlled remotely from the surgeon's console with the help of master robot manipulators. Usually, only three of the four arms are employed in head and neck surgery. They are as follows: one arm that can handle a 12-mm stereoscopic endoscope at an angle of 0° or 30° and the other two arms are equipped with 5-mm endowrist instruments[1].

Both the robotic arm instruments and the endoscope are then introduced intraorally and allow the surgeon at the console to perform procedures equivalent to conventional surgery, with the advantages of a wide range of motion with seven degrees of freedom, enhanced three-dimensional high visualization, reduction or minimal hand tremors, angled scopes help in the possibility of navigating around corners, reduction of fatigue, proper coordination of hand–eye and the possibility of telesurgery and educational opportunities to students/residents with more favorable learning techniques.

When comparing traditional open surgical approaches with TORS, it has many great advantages, such as inappropriate mandibulotomy that avoids disfigurement, it can also reduce the need for adjuvant radiotherapy and/or chemotherapy and gastrostomy/tracheostomy, improve the speech and swallowing function and reduces bleeding and postoperative pain. Quality of life (QOL) of a patient improves with minimal scarring with minimal risk of wound infection, reduced stay in hospital and time for recovery.

Surgical Setup

TORS is defined as the minimal access surgery performed via oral cavity, which uses a minimum of three robotic arms allowing for bimanual manipulation of the soft tissues of oral cavity. The surgeon's console is located at the end of the operating room, thereby allowing free space to maneuver the surgical

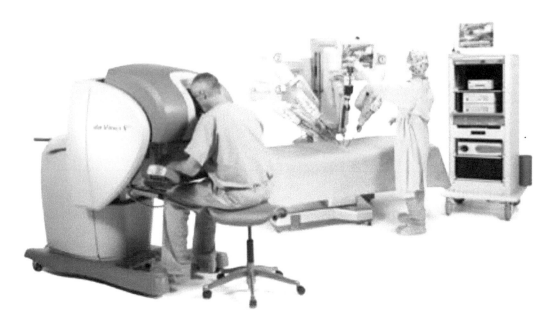

FIGURE 24.1   da Vinci robotic system.

cart that can be located on the patient's left side and is opposite to the surgeon (Figure 24.1). The assistant surgeon is placed at the head end of the patient. The anesthetic circuit and anesthesiologist are at the foot end of the patient. After induction of the patient, the scrub table and the endoscopic tower are then placed on the patient's right side. The patient is placed in a supine position strictly on the operating table. The Crow–Davis mouth gag is then placed in the oral cavity to gain surgical access and exposure and three sterile-draped robotic arms are placed in operating position. The instruments, such as atraumatic forceps along with electrocautery spatula tip, are then introduced laterally 30° from the arm supporting the 0° endoscope and placed in the left and right arms of the robot. A Feyh–Kastenbauer (FK) retractor can be used in the case of pharyngeal and laryngeal surgeries, and a flexible aspiration tube can be used for the aspiration of smoke caused by electrocautery, which is introduced into the nasopharynx through any one of the nostrils.

In skull base surgery, robotic techniques are considered the natural evolution of traditional endoscopic techniques; their role is evolving with the goal of a maximizing surgical resection of tumors by not compromising the principles of oncology of the tumor. Kupferman et al. with the help of a cadaver model reported using robotic technology to greatly facilitate the reconstruction of dura with suture on the anterior cranial base, thereby ensuring minimal trauma to critical neurovascular structures surrounding them.

As the clinical application and use of TORS for the management of HNC increases, robotically assisted reconstruction using local flaps, free flaps or primary closure holds the potential of expanding application of TORS, keeping the aim of less morbidity of the patients. The reconstruction with vascularized soft tissues into an oropharyngeal defect can thereby facilitate the improved recovery of the functions. The precision and flexibility of these arms of robot allow the placement of sutures transorally in anatomical areas of decreased accessibility and visibility with traditional open surgical techniques. Even microvascular anastomosis has been seen to prove faster and more effective with TORS. In robotic-assisted microvascular anastomosis, the robotic arms are positioned horizontally almost, in the plane of the bed, and in direct proximity of the incision given externally; while the third arm serves as a stationary assistant, micro needle preferably black diamond and nylon suture 9.0 are used for the microvascular anastomosis.

Functional Outcomes

Genden et al.[1] reported the ability to tolerate an oral diet for patients who underwent TORS at a mean of 1.4 days post surgery without any need for the placement of gastrostomy tubes. Iseli et al. reported that 83% of patients started with an oral diet within 14 days of the surgery, while 17% of those surgical patients required a feeding NG tube at 12-month follow-up, and 5.6% of these patients demonstrated signs or symptoms of aspiration. Moore et al.[2] stated that 82% of these patients were tolerating oral diet by the first visit postoperatively, whereas 17% of these patients required a feeding nasogastric tube and none of the patients required assistance with feeding at one-year follow-up. A study done by Hurtuk et al.[3] reported that 100% of the patients operated with TORS were able to take an oral diet on the day of surgery and 20% of these patients required feeding NG tubes mainly for adjuvant therapy.

Oncologic Outcomes

TORS has great oncological outcomes that are emerging slowly in the literature and they appear to be having good and promising results. In the pilot study done on 47 patients having advanced oropharyngeal SCC treated with TORS, Weinstein et al.[4] reported a 2% rate for local recurrence, a 4% regional recurrence rate and a 9% distant metastasis at a minimum period of 18-month follow-up. Overall, survival (OS) rates at 1 year were 96% and 2 years were 82%, with disease-specific survival (DFS) at 1 year was 98% and 2 years was 90%. The DFS at 1 year was 96% and 79% at 2 years of survival. Extracapsular extension (ECE) in the metastatic nodal disease was found to be statistically significant affecting the overall rate of survival, 38% of these patients avoided adjuvant chemotherapy and, due to the incidence rate of negative margins, 11% of these patients did not receive any kind of adjuvant chemoradiotherapy.

TORS provides very good and precise three-dimensional visualization and magnification in all the planes and directions, a greater freedom of instrumentation movement with tremor filtration, thereby facilitating accurate and easy surgical dissection, minimally invasive and less morbid accessibility, helping two surgeons to operate within the field. The excellent ability to control the bleeding thereby facilitates complete *en bloc resection of* tumor. Technical efficacy, feasibility and safety have been largely published by many authors in literature. In patients undergoing TORS procedure, shorter operative time and decreased length of hospital stay have been observed along with excellent functional and oncological outcomes. Good QOL with a faster recovery rate, back to normal daily routine function, allows patients to begin adjuvant therapy, if required, and is beneficial over present treatment modalities of head and neck tumors[5].

REFERENCES

1. Genden EM, Desai S, Sung CK. Transoral robotic surgery for the management of head and neck cancer: a preliminary experience. *Head & Neck*. 2009 Mar;31(3):283–9.
2. Moore EJ, Olsen KD, Martin EJ. Concurrent neck dissection and transoral robotic surgery. *Laryngoscope*. 2011 Mar;121(3):541–4.
3. Hurtuk AM, Marcinow A, Agrawal A, Old M, Teknos TN, Ozer E. Quality-of-life outcomes in transoral robotic surgery. *Otolaryngology–Head and Neck Surgery*. 2012 Jan;146(1):68–73.
4. Weinstein GS, Quon H, O'Malley Jr BW, Kim GG, Cohen MA. Selective neck dissection and deintensified postoperative radiation and chemotherapy for oropharyngeal cancer: a subset analysis of the University of Pennsylvania transoral robotic surgery trial. *Laryngoscope*. 2010 Sep;120(9):1749–55.
5. Aubry K, Yachine M, Perez AF, Vivent M, Lerat J, Scomparin A, Bessède JP. Transoral robotic surgery for head and neck cancer: a series of 17 cases. *European Annals of Otorhinolaryngology, Head and Neck Diseases*. 2011 Dec 1;128(6):290–6.

25

Perioperative Management of Head and Neck Cancer Patients

Perioperative management of head and neck cancer (HNC) patients is divided into three major categories:

1. Preoperative
2. Intraoperative
3. Postoperative

Preoperative Management

Preoperative evaluation is the most important step before making a plan for HNC patients. A proper and thorough clinical examination with a record of past medical history is required to learn of any debilitating disorders, prior to surgical procedures, etc. A proper clinical assessment of the head and neck region is done to find the primary lesion as well as the status of the neck. A clinical staging is then documented based on tumor, node, metastasis (TNM) staging called cTNM staging. Preoperative biopsy and endoscopy are performed to determine the diagnosis of the disease. Imaging, such as CT and MRI scans, is indicated based on the tissue involvement of the lesion.

A proper assessment of airway is done before the surgery by an anesthetist to anticipate any difficulty during the intubation. Routine hematological investigation is done, which includes complete blood count, screening of patients for HIV, HCV, HBsAG, liver function tests, renal function test, coagulation profile, random blood sugar levels, serum electrolytes and other required tests depending on the past medical history of the patient. Consider consultations with other specialists if a patient has any history of cardiovascular disease, diabetes; if the blood hemoglobin is below 10 g/dl, consider a whole blood transfusion. Take a written consent from the concerned specialist for surgery. A dental assessment must be done to rule out any mobile teeth, which can be risky during intubation. If there is restricted mouth opening, arrange for fiber optic laryngoscopy equipment. If there is a plan for free flap surgery, consult the plastic surgeon preoperatively and assess which flap has to be taken. A tourniquet has to be arranged for free-flap surgery and all microsurgical instruments with loupes also have to be arranged. Take high-risk consents for any anticipated risk factors intraoperatively. Explain all the risk factors to the patient and attendees before the surgery. The patient must be consoled that everything shall be fine and surgery will go well.

Intraoperative Management

The main goal of intraoperative management includes tumor resection with reconstruction based on the extent and size of the defect. The duration of the surgery might be prolonged due to the complexity of the surgery which can, in turn, increase the associated complications. Therefore, a sterile and meticulous dissection is required to decrease the risk of postoperative infection, particularly in elderly patients. Half an hour before the patient is shifted to operation room, broad-spectrum antibiotics are administered intravenously. The patient is shifted to the operating room and intubation must be smooth. Intraoperative monitoring of oxygenation, blood pressure, urine output, electrocardiogram, intravenous volume, right atrial and ventricular pressures, pulmonary artery pressure, arterial blood gases and serum electrolytes

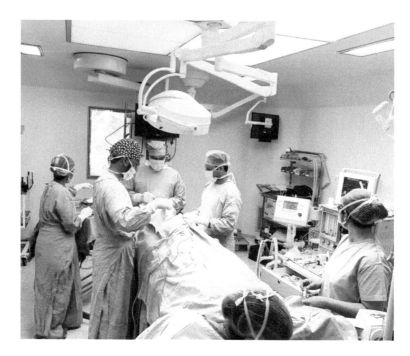

FIGURE 25.1 Operating room decorum. A good operating room, lights, fully equipped anesthetic circuit, and a highly efficient team can provide better results in perioperative management of the patient.

are done. Use of intraoperative facial nerve monitoring if required can be done. Blood transfusion or colloid transfusion must be kept ready if the preoperative blood count is low (Figure 25.1)[1].

Postoperative Management

The most important aspect in postoperative management is the nutrition of HNC patients. Approximately around 35–60% of HNC patients suffer from malnutrition, especially those who have low socioeconomic status or advanced HNCs. This is often multifactorial and may be due to tumor cachexia, dysphagia, odynophagia, dietary habits, etc. In addition, patients with HNC frequently have anorexia, early satiety and debilitation caused by prior chemotherapy and/or radiation therapy, and muscle wasting because of the increased basal metabolic rate created by tumor metabolism.

Some studies have reported that weight loss preoperatively of about 10% of total body weight is a predictive risk factor for major postoperative complications, tumor recurrence, and mortality. Mortality rates of up to 30% have been associated with 20% preoperative weight loss, and a mortality rate near 100% has been cited for 50% preoperative weight loss. Studies of clinical trials suggest that perioperative nutritional supplementation with the help of experienced dietician like protein supplements may benefit severely malnourished patients with HNC by decreasing the incidence of postoperative complications because nutritional status has a critical effect on wound healing and immune function. The enteral or parenteral route can be used and supplementation should be given for at least 10–15 days after the surgery. Nasogastric feeding tubes should be placed in patients who are unable to take adequate alimentation by mouth, although gastrostomy tubes are better tolerated. The estimated total daily caloric requirement is 25–35 kcal/kg weight, calculated on body weight and can be confirmed by dietician. The protein requirement is estimated at 2 g of protein per kilogram per day[2].

Complications of surgery postoperatively can be broadly classified into three categories—early, intermediate and late.

Immediate Complications

Hemorrhage: After surgery, the most common complication is postoperative hemorrhage. External bleeding from the surgical incision site often originates from blood vessel located subcutaneously. Often in these types of patients, direct cauterization with electrocautery or infiltration of anesthetic solution in the surrounding tissues containing epinephrine or by ligation with a free tie or nylon sutures may be done to easily control the bleeding. Persistent swelling or ballooning of the skin flaps from the surgical bed below immediately post surgery with or without any evidence of external bleeding must be attributed to a wound hematoma. Early detection of this hematoma and good working of these suctions drain without blockage, then the immediate evacuation of the accumulated blood must be done to resolve the problem. If this condition is not addressed immediately or if there is quick reaccumulation of blood, it is thereby wise to get the patient back to the operating room and surgically explore the surgical wound under strict aseptic conditions, evacuate the hematoma, identify the bleeding vessel and control it.

Airway obstruction: In patients of bilateral neck dissections for a tumor crossing midline, it may often be associated with soft tissue edema. Moreover, the primary resection of the primary upper aerodigestive malignancy may also increase the edema of the upper airway. It is always good to be prepared with all necessary surgical instruments to be carried out for a temporary elective tracheotomy to protect and maintain the airway. A surgeon must be experienced to carry out a tracheostomy.

Increased intracranial pressure: The intracranial pressure usually rises when the internal jugular vein (IJV) is ligated during neck dissection. When the ligation of one IJV is done, the pressure rises by three folds, and when both are ligated, it increases by five folds. This is usually temporary and the pressure will normalize within 24 hours. If it persists for more than 24–48 hours, head-end elevation, steroids, and mannitol are often used.

Nerve injury: The important cranial nerves that are at risk during neck dissection are the phrenic, spinal accessory, vagus, lingual, and hypoglossal nerves. Spinal accessory nerve injury causes difficulty in shrugging the shoulders called frozen shoulder syndrome and shoulder hand syndrome. Injury to hypoglossal nerve leads to a paralysis of tongue. Injury to vagus nerve may manifest as voice problems and aspiration. Injury to the phrenic nerve often causes paradoxical breathing and lingual nerve injury can cause problems in taste. Nerve injury called neuropraxia might recover within weeks to months, whereas other injuries like neurotmesis and axonotmesis have varying degrees of outcome.

Carotid sinus syndrome: This is because of undue manipulation and excess pressure on the carotid sinus baroreceptor. It may lead to bradycardia and hypotension. Postoperative scarring of tissues may also make the sinus receptor sensitive turning the head and on even palpation.

Pneumothorax: Too much lower neck dissection while resecting the level IV lymph nodes might lead to injury to the apical part of pleura and cause pneumothorax. Clinical signs of the patient may become cyanosed, restless and dyspneic after surgery. A plain radiograph of the chest most often provides the correct diagnosis. Emphysema that may be minimal might resolve itself but severe emphysema cases may require intercostal chest drains (ICD).

Intermediate Complications

Pulmonary complications: Bronchopneumonia and basal collapse are seen in patients who have the habit of smoking and have preexisting chronic obstructive lung disease.

Deep vein thrombosis: This is seen in older aged patients and involves surgeries that last for longer duration, and also in patients who are prolonged bedridden and patients with past history of pulmonary embolism, deep vein thrombosis, thrombophilia and myocardial infarction.

Chylous fistula: Thoracic duct injury often leads to chylous fistula while performing a radical neck surgery in the lower neck or mediastinum behind the IJV. If chylous fistula is suspected, every attempt should be made to suture it at the time of surgery by identifying it by head-down position and by performing modified Valsalva maneuver. It should be anticipated when the drain collection is milky in nature and increases dramatically by volume. Daily pressure dressings and fat restricted diet are the form of conservative management for chyle leak. When the drain collection reaches 600 ml per day or more, it is an absolute indication for wound re-exploration and repair of the injured thoracic duct under microscope.

Carotid artery rupture: This is usually seen when the skin wound breaks down because of previous irradiation, secondary infection and also due to patients' poor metabolic conditions. It is a fatal and deadly complication leading to immediate mortality if not intervened immediately. Control of bleeding by finger pressure immediately, airway management, blood transfusion and exploration in the operation theater has to be done.

Late Complications

- *Recurrence*: Recurrences can be at the site of primary tumor, in the lymph nodes or as a distant metastasis in lung, liver and brain
- *Lymph edema*: When the ligation of both the IJVs is done, lymphedema often follows, owing to the interruption of the lymphatic drainage channels from the head
- *Hypertrophic scars*
- *Parotid tail hypertrophy*
- *Hypothyroidism*

REFERENCES

1. Arosarena OA. Perioperative management of the head and neck cancer patient. *Journal of Oral and Maxillofacial Surgery*. 2007 Feb 1;65(2):305–13.
2. van Bokhorst-de van der Schueren MA, Quak JJ, von Blomberg-van der Flier BM, Kuik DJ, Langendoen SI, Snow GB, Green CJ, van Leeuwen PA. Effect of perioperative nutrition, with and without arginine supplementation, on nutritional status, immune function, postoperative morbidity, and survival in severely malnourished head and neck cancer patients. *American Journal of Clinical Nutrition*. 2001 Feb 1;73(2):323–32.

26

Pain Management of Locally Advanced Head and Neck Carcinomas/Palliative Care Patients

Almost 80% of head and neck patients experience pain during radiotherapy and up to 36–40% report pain even after 6 months of completion of radiotherapy. The evaluation of a patient with pain must include the following: Diagnosis of disease, prognosis of the patient, patient's goal of care, any other comorbidities and clinical symptoms, an extensive list of currently used medications for pain relief as well as comorbid conditions; past or present adherence to any medical treatments, previous experience with pain medications, cultural beliefs, spiritual dimensions, expectations of patient and family regarding pain management, socioeconomic context, insurance status, ability to obtain medications or treatment, contacts or support persons/transportation ability, medications or interventions, which are available at patient's ease.

In a study performed by Mirabile et al.[1] in 2016, 92% of head and neck patients had pain during adjuvant radiotherapy and 11% of these patients required analgesics even after 6 months of starting radiotherapy. Pain was very severe, which was also associated when the patient was in chemotherapy. Numerous local and systemic strategies are used for the management of pain due to postradiation-induced mucositis. Trotter et al. in 2013 have shown that there was not sufficient evidence in literature to recommend any ideal intervention for the management of pain in HNC. Therefore, the current protocol needs to follow the World Health Organization (WHO) Pain Ladder until further studies prove evidence otherwise and get published in literature. In a study done by Sandeep et al. in 2020, the consulting radiation oncologist had followed the WHO Pain Ladder for complications such as radiation-induced mucositis to manage the pain. There was a retrospective analysis in nature, which was dependent on data recorded by the consulting physician in a patient review chart.

Patients' assessment of pain was done by a numerical or verbal rating scale and analgesics were chosen and titrated accordingly. The assessment of pain of the patient was done two times a week and when required during management. It is done monthly after the complete treatment. There was no documentation of the pain rating scale for pain due to radiation in the review chart. The nonavailability of this pain scale was a major concern and limitation of this study. The usage of topical agents, such as gabapentin and pregabalin, was not standardized and there was a wide variation between consulting oncologists in using these topical agents. Hence, data regarding the usage of these topical agents were not analyzed.

There is less evidence of literature concerning pain management in HNC patients undergoing a systemic therapy and radiotherapy. Trotter et al.[2] had done a review on 6181 patients, which is only a single study of 30 patients, which stated that the usage of opioid was found to be 53%. The reported incidences of the use of opioid and Grade 3–4 mucositis were 53% and 23%, respectively. In the retrospective analysis of Sandeep et al., the incidence of use of opioids and Grade 3–4 mucositis is 52% and 22%, respectively. The use of strong opioids was not mentioned and is around 15% in the current study. The radiation oncologists need to quantify and identify toward the requirement of pain and analgesia of the patient during the course of radiation therapy.

WHO – Pain Relief Ladder

Step 1: Use of non-opioid (aspirin/acetaminophen), ± adjuvant,
Pain persisting or increasing, then

Step 2: Use of opioid for mild-to-moderate pain such as codeine, ± non-opioid, ± adjuvant, Pain persisting or increasing, then

Step 3: Use of opioid to moderate-to-severe pain such as morphine, ± non-opioid, ± adjuvant.

To achieve pain control, medications should be given "by the clock", that is, every 3–6 hours, rather than "on demand". This three-step approach of presenting the correct drug with the right dose at the right time is very inexpensive and effective for 80–90% of cases. Surgical intervention on appropriate painful nerves may provide further pain relief if drugs are not effective[3].

Pharmacological Options

There are three categories of pain medications (as per the WHO Pain Ladder, 1986).

Non-Opioids

Acetaminophen: It works on central nervous system and has no anti-inflammatory action. It must be the first line of the management when there is mild pain. It may be considered a good medication in addition to an opioid treatment and has been included in numerous prescribed medications. Due to the hepatic toxicity that is concerned side effect, the FDA strongly warns against the unlimited usage of such combination treatments, such as Vicodin or Percocet, with 325 mg as a maximum dosage limit of acetaminophen per dosage unit. In addition, there is a warning on the box, which highlights the potential for severe liver failure; the 1000-mg dosage must be given as per prescription only. The present maximum dosage of recommendation is 625-mg acetaminophen QID. The FDA has given 4 g daily as a maximum dosage; however, in the case of liver disease, this dosage is lowered to 2 g but only for a limited time.

NSAIDs: These drugs may have an advantage in pain that is mediated by inflammation (e.g., bone metastases, skin or musculoskeletal pain) by blocking the prostaglandin biosynthesis. The usage of these mediators is limited by their potential side effects. The most common side effects are gastrointestinal irritation, renal failure and bleeding. Recently documented risks are cardiac risks such as stroke and myocardial infarction, and hence the FDA has strengthened their existing label warning. The drugs, nowadays, that are considered to be the safest are ibuprofen and naproxen. The recommendation of these two drugs is to prescribe a short course of management from a range of 1 week to monitor closely, especially in the geriatric and cardiac patients. In certain situations, proton pump inhibitors may be considered.

The use of COX-2 selective agents, which has a reduced risk of bleeding from GI, is not often recommended in patients with palliative care. Patients requiring a proper dosage to obtain an appropriate control of pain must be increased to such a level where the side effects of these drugs are more or less similar to lower doses of nonselective NSAIDs.

Opioids

The 1986 WHO Pain Ladder, which targets cancer pain, has been a reference since a long time guiding to step up the drug from a non-opioid to a "weak" opioid if the pain did not subside, and then only to a strong one if once again, the pain control of the patient was not satisfactory. Recently, due to the usual high level of pain presented by palliative HNC patients, and based on our thorough understanding of the complex pathophysiological pain mechanisms and also with the advent of the increased number of new therapeutic formulations that are stronger, more effective opioids might be indicated earlier.

Weak

Codeine: CYP2D6 enzyme converts codeine into its active agents. Generally, 1 mg of morphine is equivalent to 10 mg of codeine. But, however, only 10% of Caucasians and 3% of Asians and African Americans have poor metabolization and will not gain benefit from these analgesic effects. Some other patients are ultrarapid metabolizers and might have an increased risk of developing any side effect. The only indication for usage of codeine is due to its action against cough, which is probably through its prodrug.

Tramadol: It is a synthetic opioid with almost five times less potency than morphine. It is not considered to be "at risk" for addiction due to its weaker action on the "mu" opioid receptors. Due to the blockage in reuptake of norepinephrine and serotonin, it may also have a benefit in addition to neuropathic pain too. But there are several certain limitations, such as with a dose of 400 mg/day, there is an increased risk of seizures in medically compromised patients, and more adverse effects than other opioids such as vomiting and nausea, commonly seen in the geriatric population. Recently, a warning was issued by the FDA regarding the risk of suicidality in a population with risk factors that are very frequent in head and neck cancer palliative care patients.

Strong

Morphine: It still remains the "gold standard" as it has been the most widely and extensively researched and studied drug and is widely available in many ranges of formulations and routes. Care must be taken in renal impairment patients due to one of its active metabolites called M3G, which may cause opioid-related toxicity.

Hydrocodone: It is slightly less potent when compared to the gold standard drug "morphine". Unfortunately, this drug is only available in combination with NSAIDs or APAP and is metabolized to hydromorphone, and the CYP 2D6 may alter the response of analgesia.

Hydromorphone: It has almost similar properties to that of morphine but has around five times more potency. It is used for parenteral use as it can be administered in smaller volumes. Similar to morphine, it also has an active metabolite called H3G, which might also lead to neurotoxicity at very high doses from impairment of renal function.

Oxycodone: It is a synthetic type of opioid and is unfortunately unavailable as parenteral formulation. It is slightly more potent than morphine (10-mg morphine = 7.5-mg oxycodone). It targets both "mu" and "kappa" receptors and this is the reason that it may have a good action on neuropathic pain and less vomiting and nausea sensation. As only 15% of this drug is excreted by the kidneys, there is a lesser risk of side effects in the case of renal failure.

Oxymorphone: It is a semisynthetic agent and two times more potent than morphine with a similar kind of side effects. It does not induce or inhibit CYP 2D6 and 3A4.

Fentanyl: It is a highly lipid-soluble opioid that can be administered parenterally, transmucosally, transdermally, intranasally, buccally, except orally. It is extremely potent, which is around 100 times stronger than the gold standard morphine, which creates safety issues.

Meperidine: It is not at all recommended because metabolites have neurotoxic effects, which increases the risk of seizures in predisposed population and also due to its high risks of addiction.

Methadone: It is a synthetic opioid. It has very poor reputation due to the variability in half-life for individuals who require optimal compliance and careful titration under guidance, its numerous cross interactions through metabolism by enzymes such as CYP3A4, 2D6 and 1A2, which increases the cardiac risks and its reputation of being a medication for "drug addicts".

Coanalgesics or Adjuvant Analgesics

These medications are not considered medications for pain but have good and relieving effects on certain types of syndromic pain such as inflammatory or neuropathic pain. Examples are antiepileptic and antidepressants drugs. Tricyclic antidepressants (TCA) are most commonly used but one must be careful of its side effects that might be related to its antimuscarinic properties. Based on the safety profile, two drugs, such as nortriptyline and desipramine, are likely better and very well tolerated with a less chance of side effects than compared to some of the other TCAs. There are numerous positive RCT-using anticonvulsants, such as gabapentin and pregabalin, for pain control as well. They are less effective than TCAs but have a better side-effect profile and are not metabolized hepatically. The co-analgesic presenting a very good efficacy level in neuropathic pain with the least side effect is gabapentin.

Corticosteroids have been indicated in various situations where inflammation is the leading cause of the syndromic pain such as cerebral edema, neuropathic pain, spinal cord compression, visceral pain or bone. High-dose steroids are used in certain conditions; however, ongoing treatment should be avoided due to their major side effects.

Reliable access to strong opioids, such as morphine, is necessary to deliver quality palliative care in locally advanced cases that are surgically unresectable and recurrent tumors, a key component of global cancer control. Despite its approval or importance as a WHO essential medicine, morphine is very limited or absent in many low- and middle-income countries, such as India. This problem is significant as 60% of the world's cancer mortality occurs in low- and middle-income countries and 80–85% of patients in these countries present with advanced- or late-stage diseases, mostly left with palliative care option.

There are some barriers regarding opioid availability due to its scarce availability, restrictive laws, regulations and licensing requirements that drastically limit the distribution of controlled substances and medical decision-making of providers.

Opioid consumption data indicate that developed and higher income source countries consume a disproportionate amount of morphine for medicinal purposes when compared with low- and middle-income countries. However, there are certain regions in India, which have made tremendous progress in developing palliative care services with limited access to morphine. Among 2.4 million people in India suffering from cancer, around 1.6 million are likely to be in pain and only 0.4% of the Indian population could benefit from opioid therapy and can thus access the opioid medication[3].

REFERENCES

1. Mirabile A, Airoldi M, Ripamonti C, Bolner A, Murphy B, Russi E, et al. Pain management in head and neck cancer patients undergoing chemo-radiotherapy: clinical practical recommendations. *Critical Reviews in Oncology/Hematology*. 2016;99:100–6.
2. Trotter PB, Norton LA, Loo AS, Munn JI, Voge E, Ah-See KW, et al. Pharmacological and other interventions for head and neck cancer pain: a systematic review. *Journal of Oral & Maxillofacial Research*. 2013;3:e1.
3. LeBaron V, Beck SL, Maurer M, Black F, Palat G. An ethnographic study of barriers to cancer pain management and opioid availability in India. *Oncologist*. 2014 May;19(5):515.

Index

Note: Locators in *italics* represent figures.

T - #0192 - 111024 - C45 - 254/178/8 - PB - 9780367421311 - Gloss Lamination